CW00766453

a peek into

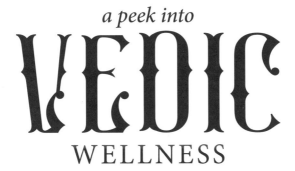

VEDIC

WELLNESS

by

Vishnupriya Thacker

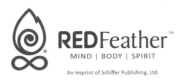

REDFeather™

MIND | BODY | SPIRIT

An Imprint of Schiffer Publishing, Ltd.

Copyright © 2022 by Vishnupriya Thacker

Library of Congress Control Number: 2021942743

Edited by James Young
Designed by Christopher Bower
Cover design by Brenda McCallum
Type set in Philosopher / Minion Pro

ISBN: 978-0-7643-6369-6
Printed in India

Published by REDFeather Mind, Body, Spirit
An imprint of Schiffer Publishing, Ltd.
4880 Lower Valley Road
Atglen, PA 19310
Phone: (610) 593-1777; Fax: (610) 593-2002
Email: Info@schifferbooks.com
Web: www.redfeathermbs.com

For our complete selection of fine books on this and related subjects, please visit our website at www.schifferbooks.com. You may also write for a free catalog.

Schiffer Publishing's titles are available at special discounts for bulk purchases for sales promotions or premiums. Special editions, including personalized covers, corporate imprints, and excerpts, can be created in large quantities for special needs. For more information, contact the publisher.

We are always looking for people to write books on new and related subjects. If you have an idea for a book, please contact us at proposals@schifferbooks.com.

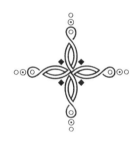

Contents

Acknowledgments

I am grateful to the Universe/Paramatma for the inspiration to create this introductory book. During the process, I was blessed with support from some incredible people and extend my heartfelt gratitude to my family and friends.

I would like to give a special note of appreciation to my close friend and respected *Ayurvedacharya* Dr. A. Bapat for her medical contribution, guidance, and expert Ayurvedic knowledge.

Additionally, I would like to clarify that I am an Ayurvedic wellness and spiritual-healing coach (not an Ayurvedic doctor), and an avid practitioner of this age-old science along with spirituality (both general and Vedic). I am passionate about this subject and have illustrated the important concepts in the following sections, after imbibing and practicing many of the principles in my own personal journey to my I AM. Thank you.

Namaste and love,

Vishnupriya

Introduction

My dear readers,

This book is to introduce you to the basic concepts of Ayurveda, Vedic wellness, *and spirituality. The book has been divided into ten sections and has been designed in a question-and-answer format to make the reading experience easier and pleasurable.*

I was inspired to write this book when I was explaining to a business acquaintance what I do as an Ayurvedic Wellness and Spiritual Healing coach. He was intrigued, wanted to know more, and undertook his own research. A couple of weeks later, I received a phone call from him, during which he suggested that I write about basic concepts on this topic that would make it easier for a potential student of ancient wisdom or a reader to understand.

I would like to dedicate this book to both my grandmothers and my mother as a token of gratitude for all that I have learned from them. It is from my maternal grandmother that I imbibed the appreciation for exotic healing spices and my initial training in Indian cuisine, which was further imparted to me by my mother.

My paternal grandmother contributed to the growth of my personality, since she often recited life stories that were inspiring, and on occasion provided some gems of wisdom—a few of which came from the spiritual books that she enjoyed reading.

I have truly enjoyed writing this book with the grace of Paramatma. My earnest wish is that you appreciate my initial attempt at explaining some concepts of ancient Vedic wisdom that have been left to us by our predecessors as an invaluable gift.

Namaste and love,
Vishnupriya

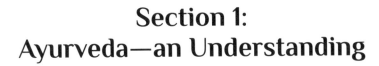

Section 1:
Ayurveda—an Understanding

What is Ayurveda?

Ayurveda is an ancient, 5,000-year-old, well-balanced science of medicine from India. It is a healing science that centers on the alignment of mind, body, and soul, with a focus on one's goals in life, diet (including the use of herbs and spices), exercise, spiritual growth, and overall lifestyle. The aim of Ayurveda is maintenance, prevention, and healing, which is why it is also known to be the science for the longevity of life. This ancient science of medicine propounds that for better physical, mental, emotional, and spiritual health, one must learn to live in accordance with the rhythms of nature.

It describes the four aims of life as

- **Dharma**: duty or righteousness
- **Artha**: wealth
- **Kama**: desire or love
- **Moksha**: salvation

What is the origin of Ayurveda?

The origins of Ayurveda date back to 6000 BCE, when it began as an oral tradition that was passed on by sages in the ancient Vedic culture. Ayurveda is attributed to Lord Dhanvantri, who was the physician to the gods and who received this gift from Lord Brahma, as stated in Hindu mythology. It is one of the oldest systems of medicine in the world. The first recorded medical text of Ayurveda originates from the Vedas, especially the *Atharva Veda*.

The main Ayurvedic classical texts are:

Charaka Samhita: which was written in Sanskrit by Charaka, the father of Ayurveda at the ancient University of Takshila, around 800 BCE and is a compilation of medical theory and practice.[1]

Sushruta Samhita: which was written in Sanskrit by Sushruta around 700 BCE and details the definition of health, *Marma* points (junctures of *Prana* or vital life force), and reconstructive surgery.[1]

Ashtanga Sangraha and ***Ashtanga Hridaya***: which was written in poetry and prose form, respectively, in Sanskrit around 400 BCE by Vaghabhatta, an Ayurvedic physician, who stressed the *material value of life*.[1]

How far and wide did Ayurveda spread?

In ancient times, the wisdom of the Vedic sciences and Ayurveda spread to Indonesia, Burma, Tibet in the East, and to Greece in the West. The Buddhists were the early adopters of this knowledge. Today, Ayurveda is quickly spreading across the globe and contributing to the synthesis of Eastern and Western medicine. It is being accepted readily as a source for mind-body-spirit integration, and its knowledge is being harnessed for the longevity of life and overall well-being.

What is Ayurvedic wisdom based on?

Ayurvedic wisdom is based on the six Vedic schools of philosophy. These schools and their founders are

- **Yoga**: Patanjali[2]
- **Sankhya**: Kapila[2]
- **Vaisheshika**: Kanada[2]
- **Nyaya**: Gautam[2]
- **Purva Mimansa**: Jaimini[2]
- **Vedanta**: Vyasa[2]

Sankhya, Nyaya, and *Vaisheshika* are the application of numbers, precision, logic,[2] and rationality, in their approach to objects and categorization in dealing with the external world.

Purva Mimansa expounds the importance of duty and dharma as stated in the Vedas[2] and Upanishads (Vedic texts). It advances the wisdom of the ancient scriptures through mantras and the experience of truth, which in itself is all encompassing.

Vedanta focuses on the spiritual themes of the Vedas—the nature of the Absolute Brahman[2] and the unconditioned Self or Higher Consciousness. This philosophy propounds that the Divine exists in every living being as the Atman and the oneness of existence. The Atman is beyond birth and death and is not affected by the body or our fluctuating thoughts or the mind. The Atman is one with the Brahman or Paramatma. The objective in life is to explore one's spirituality, to connect with Higher Consciousness or I AM, and to manifest our divinity.

Yoga, written by Patanjali, describes Yoga practices that can be traced back to the Vedas, with a focus on Raja Yoga, emphasizing devotional practices, meditation, and renunciation.

In short, the Purva Mimansa, Vedanta, and Yoga schools of philosophy focus on our inner growth and how we can evolve spiritually.

What are the five elements in Ayurveda?

Ayurveda explains that we are all connected to nature and other living beings. The five elements of nature, known as the *Panchamahabhutas*, are:

- *Prithvi*: earth
- *Jala*: water
- *Vayu*: air
- *Akash* or *Antariksha*: space
- *Agni*: fire

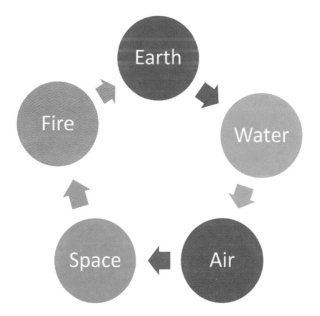

What are the characteristics of these five elements?

- *Prithvi* is solid and stable.
- *Jala* is liquid and changing.
- *Vayu* is mobile and dynamic.
- *Agni* is hot and transformative.
- *Akash* is expansive and has the ability to fill.

What can we learn from nature as described in the Vedic texts?

Earth is stable, grounding, comforting and holds everyone with equal support. We can learn from the earth to accept and respect everyone on an equal basis.

A tree teaches us about the oneness of life and interconnectedness. A leaf cannot fall from a tree without the existence of the tree itself, which exists in the ground due to the earth in which it is rooted, and in turn, the earth exists because of this planet, which is an integral part of this universe.

The sun provides us with light and energy, bringing with it the dawn of a new day. Every day we can imbibe from the sun the important message that there is a light after darkness, and with it comes a plethora of opportunities raising hope in the world. On an emotional level, all of us go through cycles, similar to the rhythms in nature. So, if you feel low one day, then know that just like the sun rises the next day, bringing with it new hope, likewise you can also begin the next day with aspirations and positivity.

The beautiful night sky with its multitude of stars reminds us that we are not alone but part of a global community where we all can shine our individual beauty and light.

Water from a river can flow and merge into the ocean without changing its essential form. Similarly, each one of us may come from different backgrounds, cultures, and beliefs, and yet what binds us all together is that we are all connected, since we come from the same Source. We are all one!

Why is Ayurveda considered to be a holistic medical system?

A doctor in Ayurveda, or *Ayurvedacharya* or an Ayurvedic holistic health coach, is not only concerned with the physical body during a diagnosis, but will also take into consideration the patient's emotional and mental state, lifestyle, food habits, sleep and dream patterns, childhood, daily habits, and long-held beliefs or issues.

In short, before prescribing a treatment, a pulse diagnosis along with a full understanding of the physical, psychological, and emotional condition is conducted, making Ayurveda a holistic science of medicine that focuses on mind-body-spirit.

What are the various subject areas in the Ayurvedic medicinal system?

Ayurveda is divided into eight subject areas or sections of medicine called *Astanga Ayurveda*, which include:

Kaya Chikitsa or **general or internal medicine**: patient evaluation; also covers healing and cleansing routines known as *Panchakarma*.

Shalya Tantra or **surgery**: removal of obstructions.

Shalakya Tantra or **ENT and ophthalmology**: healing the diseases of the ear, nose, and throat.

Agad Tantra or **toxicology**: removal of toxic poisons from the physical system.

Kaumar Bhritya Balchikitsa or **pediatrics**: covers children's ailments, pre- and postnatal care.

Bhoot Vidya Graha Chikitsa or **psychology and psychiatry**: all aspects of mental health and psychiatric medicine. Treatments such as meditation and *Pranayama* (breathing techniques) are suggested for relaxation.

Rasayana or **rejuvenation therapies**: this covers all rejuvenating measures, including *Abhayanga* or massage treatment.

Vajikarna or **aphrodisiac therapy**: This therapy targets sexual health and fertility treatments. The aspects of Tantra are considered to be a method for spiritual growth, to provide an understanding of Shiva and Shakti energies, and to strengthen the intimate bond between partners.

What are the suggested treatments in Ayurveda?

Ayurveda takes into consideration bio-individuality; however, the general treatments suggested by an *Ayurvedacharya* (Ayurvedic doctor) or Ayurvedic/holistic health coach are:

- Diet and lifestyle choices
- Exercise
- Sleep
- Meditation

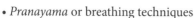

- *Pranayama* or breathing techniques
- *Panchakarma* or detox and cleansing therapies
- *Rasayana* or rejuvenation methods
- Spiritual healing

What are the fundamental components of the body according to Ayurveda?

The fundamental components of the body are the:

Doshas: the three physical and psychological Doshas. Physically, the Doshas are *Vata*, *Pitta*, and *Kapha*. The psychological Doshas are *Sattva*, *Rajas*, and *Tamas*.

Dhatus: the seven tissue elements; namely, plasma or *Rasa*, blood or *Rakta*, muscle or *Mamsa*, adipose tissue or fat or *Medha*, bones or *Asthi*, bone marrow or *Majja*, and hormones or *Shukra*.

Malas: the three waste products; namely, urine or *Mutra*, stool or *Sakht*, and sweat or *Swedha*.

Agni: the "digestive fire" is an extremely important consideration in Ayurveda. It is responsible for the transformation of food into energy, metabolism, healthful life span, and overall immunity of the individual.

What are the physical *Doshas* and *Prakruti* in Ayurveda?

Dosha is the physiological force in the body, and constitution or *Prakruti* is a combination of three physical Doshas (*Vata*, *Pitta*, *Kapha*), with two being in dominance in most individuals.

Prakruti is the *unique makeup* of a person—physically it covers one's body structure, body frame, skin condition, hair texture, and facial features. Psychologically it refers to traits that a person has—whether he is fearful and anxious or bold and brave, for example, and functionally it includes skills, talents, and the potentiality of the individual.

What are the characteristics of the physical Doshas?

Vata: Vata individuals have a thin body structure, eyes of differing sizes, fair strength, and a tendency toward dryness in the skin and hair. They tend to learn quickly, are creative, make friends easily, are somewhat impatient, and tend to have fluctuating thoughts.

Pitta: Pitta individuals have a medium, proportionate body structure, sharp features, and shiny skin and hair. They tend to make friends related to their profession, are goal-oriented, speak coherently, have adequate strength and good memory, and tend to lean towards perfection.

Kapha: Kapha individuals have a broad, plump body frame, excellent strength, and thick hair. They have long-lasting friends and strong family relationships, have sweet and slow communication, and are generous, loving in nature, and slow to learn new things.

Doshas

Vata: comprises air and space
Pitta: comprises fire and water
Kapha: comprises earth and water

What are the characteristics of the psychological Doshas?
Sattvic mindset: Individuals with a Sattvic mindset are intelligent, disciplined, calm, compassionate, positive, spiritual minded, honest, respectful, have good memory, and see life as a continuous learning process.

Sattvic individuals are dedicated to their work and profession. They see this as creative endeavors, which are carried out with true integrity with the intention that it is best surrendered to Higher Consciousness with trust and faith. It is their duty to do the work as an offering to the *Supreme* with full humility.

Illustration

Meet Sarah, a music school teacher, who is passionate about teaching music and encouraging her students to practice in order to increase their skills on the musical instruments of their choice. Sarah is dedicated to her duty—she goes above and beyond to ensure that their talents are nurtured, provides them with positive, constructive feedback, and is selfless in giving them additional time. The twenty talented students in Sarah's music class, in turn, genuinely appreciate her efforts, look forward to learning from her, and consider her to be their favorite teacher.

Rajasic mindset: Individuals with a Rajasic mindset are creative, dynamic, brave, and ambitious; like power and authority; are go-getters, proud, distracted at times, competitive; and can be selfish. These individuals are very creative, have great ideas, and like to implement them; however, they are usually very concerned with achieving their own goals and dreams. They like opulence, parties, good food, and being socially visible.

Illustration

Meet Sameer, a hardworking advertising executive, who is very creative and designs unique and effective ad campaigns. He has been with the agency for the past ten years. The owner of the company totally supports Sameer since he is the top employee, who not only is a perfectionist at his work but also knows how to manage client relationships. The HR department has, however, received complaints about Sameer being controlling of his team members and a bit abrasive at times.

Tamasic mindset: Individuals with a Tamasic mindset have unknown fears and anxiety; can become disrespectful of others, selfish, and lazy; are less inclined toward hard work; are complainers; and do not put effort toward improving their lives or changing their lifestyle. They like to enjoy the benefits that are given to them, without any real inclination toward taking responsibility for themselves and others.

Illustration

Meet Paul, a maintenance technician who has been out of a job for the past two years. He complains when he finds employment, becomes tired of his work routine, and leaves suddenly. After losing each position he returns to his parents' home to live, but does not take on any responsibility. Paul's parents are tired of his impulsive lifestyle and don't know how to encourage their lazy son to make constructive life changes. They are worried about his future—that he will never be able to consistently hold a job going forward or change his ways to become stable and responsible.

What are the imbalances of the physical Doshas?

Vata: aggravated or imbalanced Vata can result in restlessness, fear, anxiety, lowered immunity, reduced life span, stiffness in the joints, tiredness, and tremors.

Pitta: variance in Pitta in the body can result in increased acidity, heart-burn, digestive issues, negative emotions such as anger, and a quicker transformation, which results in speeding up the aging process.

Kapha: aggravated Kapha can result in diseases such as high cholesterol, weight gain, heart disease, arthritis, congestion in the chest and lungs, instability, envy, and greed.

What are the functions of the three *doshic* energies in the body?

Vata: Vata energy in the body is responsible for breathing, pulsation, the passage of food, excretion, and peristalsis. Vata activates every action and the senses in the body. It controls both our sensory and motor organs along with the respiratory, circulatory, gastrointestinal, and excretory movements.

Vata is predominantly located in the large intestine, thighs, feet, bones, skin, ears, and urinary bladder.

Pitta: Pitta energy is *fire* energy, which makes it responsible for the generation of heat, transformation in the body, and the conversion of food into energy that affects our immunity and life span. It specifically helps us with digestion, absorption, skin color, body temperature, intelligence, vision, bravery, and comprehension.

Pitta is predominantly located in the stomach, skin, eyes, hormones, blood, liver, spleen, and gallbladder.

Kapha: Kapha energy protects the organs and forms the preservative fluids in the body. It is responsible for the process of cohesion, maintaining the structure of the body, and providing nutrition to the tissues or *Dhatus*. We gain our strength and stability due to Kapha energies, which help increase our immunity, build our tissues, and contribute to our intelligence and memory.

Kapha is predominantly in the chest, throat, sinuses, nose, stomach, joints, and preservative fluids in the body, such as plasma and the cerebrospinal fluid.

What are the lifestyle suggestions for the three physical Doshas?

Vata: Vata individuals can feel restless and agitated when imbalanced. In order to counter this, Ayurveda makes the following suggestions:

- Ensure that you have a consistent routine.
- Exercise daily by walking for 30 minutes.
- Establish a morning meditation practice for each day.
- Get a lot of rest as needed.

Pitta: Pitta individuals find it difficult to detach when they are involved in a project or at work, which can result in feeling pressured. In order to counter this, Ayurveda advises the following:

- Try to balance your day—remain cool and calm mentally, emotionally, and physically.
- Avoid the midday sun, heat, and steam.
- Exercise during the cooler part of the day, and water sports such as swimming are preferable.

Kapha: Kapha people can become bored or lethargic, which results in lowering their metabolism, causing both physical and mental imbalances. In order to counter this, Ayurveda instructs the following:

- Exercise on a daily basis. Keep active. Do exercises that really push you, such as jogging, martial arts, and racquetball.
- Take hot baths or steam inhalations consistently to avoid congestion, especially during spring, fall, and winter months.
- Have variety in your day and do not take daytime naps.
- Include a new experience in your life on a regular basis, such as meeting new people or trying out a new activity or hobby.

Why is good sleep recommended in Ayurveda?

Good sleep is essential for increasing *Ojas* or immunity and provides relaxation to the mind and body. A lack of proper sleep is not beneficial for the body and overall health—it results in headache, body ache, lethargy, and a burning sensation in the eyes. If you do not get enough sleep, it could affect your food intake, which has a resultant effect on the proper functioning and the regularity of your bowel movements.

There are some indications of poor sleep, as below:

- It is when you have disturbed sleep at night.
- You wake up in the morning with body soreness or a headache (or both).
- In the morning when you rise, you feel tired instead of feeling fresh.
- You are not alert throughout the day, which affects your overall productivity.

According to Ayurveda, sleeping on the left side (which opens up the right nostril) is the best position to ensure that digestion, absorption, and assimilation are proper. This prevents heartburn and other digestive issues. Sleeping on the left side also prevents snoring (if your head is slightly tilted on a pillow sideways), helps with better elimination, facilitates lymphatic drainage, relieves back pain, and promotes better functioning of the heart. Sleeping on the stomach is not recommended at all, since it disturbs the digestive system and normal breathing patterns. In the ancient texts it is suggested to sleep with your head toward the south or east to increase your energy and well-being.

If you face any difficulty going to bed or getting sleep at night, a cup of hot turmeric milk (recipe provided in the "Fun with Spices" section) is suggested.

What does Ayurveda recommend for establishing a daily routine?

Ayurveda recommends a daily routine so as to establish balance in life. This structure contributes to our physical, mental, emotional, and spiritual health. This is known as *Dinacharya* and includes the following:

- Waking up daily on time.
- Drinking water just after you awake—warm water is preferable to remove any toxins that have accumulated from the previous day.
- Cleaning your teeth, gargling with warm water, doing a tongue cleanse (using a tongue scraper), and doing an oil pulling.
- Meditating and saying a short prayer.
- Exercising to get your energy levels going.
- Doing an oil self-massage before having a bath.
- Giving thanks and showing gratitude to Paramatma before starting your day's activities with a smile.

What are the Ayurvedic detox therapies or treatments that are suggested for overall wellness?

The five detox (*Panchakarma*) therapies in Ayurveda are:

Abhayanga or **body (tissue) massage**: herbal oils are used and massaged into the entire body to release toxins from the tissue layers, improve the body's immunity and circulation, and lubricate the joints. This, in turn, improves sleep and calms down the nervous system. An effective Ayurvedic massage method is to heat a cloth bundle *potli* that contains herbs and oil, and then apply it to the body muscles and tissues.

Shirodhara or **herbal oil flow**: herbal oil that is continuously streamed onto your forehead as a means to reduce stress. The added benefits are relaxation, better memory, sight, and hearing.

Nasya or **nasal therapy**: putting herbal oil drops in the nasal passages with the use of a neti pot helps prevent hair loss and wrinkles and sharpens the sense organs.

Basti or **herbal enema**: herbal oil that is part of an enema treatment to remove toxins from the colon. This therapy is great for dealing with fatigue, constipation, or sexual disorders but is not suggested for those who suffer from shortness of breath or anemia.

Swedana or **body heating**: application of heat to various parts of the body to melt the toxins and allow them to release as sweat through the skin. This method helps increase blood circulation and enhances skin elasticity.

In addition to the above therapies, there are a few other recommendations from Ayurveda for every morning. These include:

Tongue scraping: use a stainless-steel tongue scraper to remove any toxic residue or white coating on your tongue.

Oil pulling: use coconut or sesame oil and swish the oil in the mouth for a few minutes to remove any toxic buildup. (*Discard the oil from the mouth into the trash can instead of the basin so as to avoid any inconvenience caused by the discarded oil, which can clog the basin pipes.*)

Hot water intake: consume hot or room-temperature water first thing in the morning after waking and before each meal, since this helps cleanse the body and activate the digestive fire or *Agni*.

What is *Ojas* in Ayurveda?

Ojas: Means the immunity and vitality of the body. A person who has a healthy Ojas will have a balanced digestion and lifestyle; will radiate energy from the inside out; will have shiny hair and skin, increased energy, bright and shiny eyes, and a peaceful disposition, with the ability to handle any kind of stress; and will be generous at heart. The quality of one's Ojas is related to the strength of the digestive fire or *Agni* within the individual.

Section 2:
Ayurvedic Nutrition

In practically every culture in the world, food is a predominant component. Food becomes an essential part of family get-togethers, celebrations, and social or professional gatherings. It provides us with sustenance and comfort. In most homes, the kitchen or the dining room becomes the center for discussions bringing all the family members together—whether it is a new culinary dish that excites the palette or simply enjoying slices of fresh seasonal fruit. It is therefore crucial that we focus on the kind of food that we consume.

The quality of mind and body is affected by the kinds of food that we appreciate and ingest. In this regard, Ayurveda states that foods can be *Sattvic, Rajasic*, and *Tamasic*. There are also six tastes that are recommended for each meal—*sweet, sour, salty, bitter, astringent,* and *pungent*.

What are Sattvic, Rajasic, and Tamasic foods?

Foods contain a certain *Prana* or energy that has a pre- and postdigestive impact on our bodies, once consumed.

Sattvic foods: are pure and are full of life-force energy that imparts a feeling of balance, love, kindness, harmony, lightness, contentment, and clarity in the body. These are usually healthful foods such as organic fresh vegetables, fruits, unprocessed grains, nuts, and seeds. Food that is freshly prepared, tasty, easy to digest, and packed with nourishing nutrients is considered Sattvic in nature.

Rajasic foods: are hot, spicy, and salty. These foods tend to tempt us and stimulate our senses. Once consumed, they can rouse us to action, the desire to create, and also cause some negative tendencies such as agitation, anger, irritation, and jealousy. Some examples of Rajasic foods are pickles, tamarind, sour cream, and nightshade vegetables.

Tamasic foods: are those that develop a feeling of fullness once we finish our meals, leading to lethargy and resistance. These foods can be grounding in nature but can also quickly induce a sense of dullness or sleep. Stored, stale foods are referred to as Tamasic since they do not contain the same level of nutrients or energy as when they were freshly prepared. Some examples of Tamasic foods are red meat, pork, beef, heavy cheese or cream, and sweets.

How does nature teach us to eat?

Ayurveda advises us to flow with the rhythms of nature, and it is recommended to eat fresh foods that are in season. In the heat of the summer months, for example, consume foods that have a predominance of water, such as watermelon, lychee, orange, zucchini, and cucumber. In the cold winter months, we need more grounding foods, such as bananas, apples, squash, and sweet potato.

What is the advice from Ayurveda on how we should eat meals?

Ayurveda advocates being immersed in enjoying your meal with awareness and gratitude. Sit and eat your food in a calm environment, without watching television or discussing controversial topics at the dinner table. If you are lucky to have food to eat, do so after thanking Paramatma (Divine/Pure Consciousness) and wish for the same blessing for all in the world. Ayurveda advises us to consume food with all our senses in order to enjoy the meal fully. Eat good, fresh food that is pleasing to all the five senses—touch, sight, taste, smell, and sound. This is called eating mindfully and being present in the moment during meal times.

See the illustration below:

Pick Up an Apple . . .

Does it look bright red, making your mouth water?
When you hold it in your hand to bite, does it feel nice and smooth in your fingers?
Does it smell fresh and not old or stale?
When you eat it, does it taste sweet and delicious?
When you bite into it, do you hear the crunch of the apple?

What is digestive fire and why is it important?

Agni or digestive fire is very important in Ayurveda, since it is considered to be the cause of good health or disease in the body. If Agni is strong yet balanced, or *Sthayi*, then digestion will be smooth and stable, resulting in increased immunity and energy. This in turn fosters a long and healthy life.

If Agni becomes weak or deficient, or *Kasaya*, in the body, due to diet or lifestyle choices, then there will be the creation of toxins, or *Ama*, making the body imbalanced and causing physical and mental ailments. The Agni can be further weakened due to emotional issues that the person is dealing with.

An excess, or *Vriddhi*, of Agni also becomes a problem since it increases the rate of transformation in the body, causing imbalance and speeding up the aging process.

It is suggested to avoid consuming ice-cold water because it dampens the digestive fire. Instead, make it a habit to drink room-temperature or warm water, especially when you wake up in the morning. The consumption of warm or room-temperature water first thing in the morning will aid in flushing your body of toxins and cause your internal organs to energize, without having to be dependent on caffeine or sugar. Some people tend to have a better sleep if they consume room-temperature water before going to bed. Try this out for yourself, and if you find it beneficial, include this practice in your daily routine.

What is *Vipaka*?

In Ayurveda, digestion and Agni are the most important aspects to be considered for optimum health, and *Vipaka* is closely related to this. Vipaka is the postdigestive energy in the body that affects the quality of the tissues once the food has been digested in the gastrointestinal tract, depending on the strength of the digestive Agni. If you have a strong Agni, the energy being produced will be good for the tissues, resulting in a strong mind, emotions, and physical body.

What are the suggestions for balancing the physical Doshas?

Ayurveda has suggested some general guidelines for balancing the three main physical Doshas:

Vata:

- Do not skip meals.
- Consume warm, cooked, and grounding food.
- Avoid frozen, raw, and overprocessed food.
- Include warming spices such as ginger, garlic, and red chili powder, and especially those spices that stimulate digestion.
- Consume whole grains, since these are nourishing and grounding.
- Cooked mung beans are recommended for Vata since they are easier to digest than other pulses or beans, which can cause constipation.
- Seasonal fruits are good for Vata in general but should be consumed in moderation.
- Include steamed or lightly cooked vegetables.
- Eat nuts and seeds that are lightly roasted and taken in moderation.
- Consume dairy products such as cow's milk, goat's milk, cheese, butter, and ghee.
- Animal products are acceptable except for red meat and pork.

Tastes to balance *Vata*:

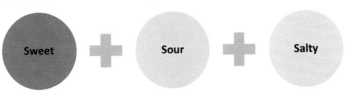

Pitta:

- Do not wait until you are very hungry, or skip meals.
- Avoid consuming too much oil.
- Most grains are good for strength except buckwheat, rye, teff, and millet.
- Pitta has a good digestive fire to digest most beans and dairy products.
- Fruits that are cooling and decrease thirst are recommended.
- Most vegetables can be digested by Pitta, but deep frying or using too much oil should be avoided while cooking them.
- Nuts and seeds such as pecans, cashews, and sesame are not recommended.
- Animal products in general should be avoided, except for chicken, turkey, and freshwater fish.
- Reduce your salt intake.
- Have cooling spices such as coriander, mint, and cumin.
- Increase your intake of cool, healthful, and light foods to balance Pitta.

Tastes to balance Pitta:

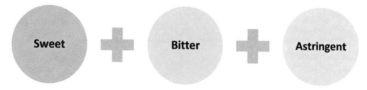

Sweet ✚ Bitter ✚ Astringent

Kapha:

- Do not skip meals.
- Drink hot or warm water throughout the day.
- Avoid heavy, sweet, oily, and fatty food.
- Eat light and dry food. (*Please consult an Ayurvedacharya or Ayurvedic coach if you are in Vata age.*)
- Grains are to be consumed in moderation.
- Beans are a good protein source for Kapha.
- Dairy products contribute to congestion and are better avoided. However, buttermilk and goat's milk or skim milk yogurt may be consumed in moderation.
- Eat fruits in moderation.
- Most vegetables are good and can be taken raw in the summer months.

- Eat nuts and seeds in a balanced manner. (Too much can result in congestion.)
- Include spices such as red chili, black pepper, ginger, and basil in your dishes.
- White and lean meat is preferable.

Tastes to balance *Kapha*:

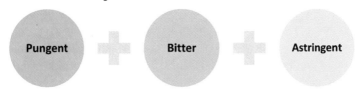

What are the healthful foods that are good for Vata, Pitta, and Kapha according to Ayurveda?

Fruits that balance Vata

apricots, avocado, ripe bananas, cantaloupe, cherries, figs, papaya, oranges, peaches, pears, plums, raspberries, and strawberries

Vegetables that balance Vata

beets, carrots, mustard greens, okra, squash, sweet potato, yams, green beans, peppers, and eggplant

Fruits that balance Pitta

apples, avocado, blueberries, cantaloupe, cranberries, dates, figs, raspberries, strawberries, and pineapple

Vegetables that balance Pitta

asparagus, bean sprouts, artichokes, brussels sprouts, cabbage, cauliflower, kale, lettuce, cucumber, mushrooms, squash, zucchini, and peas

Fruits that balance Kapha

apples, cherries, dry fruits, cranberries, raisins, pomegranate, prunes, grapefruit, and oranges

Vegetables that balance Kapha

asparagus, green beans, brussels sprouts, cabbage, cauliflower, celery, kale, lettuce, mustard greens, spinach, turnips, red radish, and daikon (white) radish

A plate of food that has fresh vegetables and fruits and that is in keeping with the cycles of nature or the seasons (with varied colors), and covering the six tastes, can become very appealing to our senses.

Grains that balance Vata

rice, quinoa (in moderation), cooked oats, wheat, barley, and amaranth

Nuts and seeds that balance Vata

cashews, sunflower seeds, pumpkin seeds, sesame seeds, almonds, walnuts, peanuts (all of them are best roasted and not raw)

Grains that balance Pitta

basmati/brown rice, cooked oats, wheat, barley, amaranth, tapioca, granola, and quinoa (in moderation)

Nuts and seeds that balance Pitta

walnuts, almonds (soaked), pistachios, sunflower seeds, pumpkin seeds, and coconut

Grains that balance Kapha

rye, millet, buckwheat, corn, barley, quinoa, muesli, tapioca, and granola

Nuts and seeds that balance Kapha

sunflower seeds, pumpkin seeds, flaxseed, walnuts, and cashews (in moderation)

In summary, what does Ayurveda suggest about food consumption?

Ayurveda advises that food must be consumed with complete focus and in a calm environment. Food tastes better if we can offer gratitude prior to consuming our meal, and eating mindfully. It is preferable if food is eaten fresh and is attractive to all the five senses.

It is recommended to chew each morsel about 32 times, and the stomach should be filled—one-third with food, one-third with water, and one-third with air. Ayurveda says that the amount of food in each meal that is really needed for your body is an *Anjali*, or two open palms held close together, and does not require more than that.

After your meal, sit quietly for a few minutes and avoid any physical activity that can disturb the process of digestion.

In addition to the above, there are some guidelines recommended for those wanting to follow an Ayurvedic dietary lifestyle:

- Include foods with the six tastes in each meal.
- Foods should be consumed with balanced attributes. Example: A meal should consist both of heavy and light foods, as well as warm or cool food items.
- Have Sattvic-rich foods that increase the positive energy in the physical, mental, and emotional bodies. Foods such as almonds, honey, mung beans, and fresh vegetables and fruits are considered to be Sattvic in nature.
- Buy fresh, organic, and seasonal foods for your daily meals rather than processed foods. It is suggested to buy cooling foods such as watermelon and cucumber, which are abundant in the summer season.
- Make your meals appealing to all the senses and include variety. If the plate is appetizing through color, flavor, aroma, and texture, then you will be more fulfilled and will prevent overeating.
- Include spices and herbs while cooking food for your meals, since they have healing benefits and enhance digestion.

What are the different foods that can be categorized by the six tastes (*Rasa*)?
Ayurveda suggests having food with all six tastes on your plate—sweet, sour, salty, bitter, astringent, and pungent. As an example, if your plate contains potato, cheese, salted nuts, rhubarb, and raspberries, you would have covered the sweet, sour, salty, pungent, bitter, and astringent tastes, respectively.

The concept of the six tastes becomes interesting once we understand what each is composed of. Sweet or *Madhura* consists of earth and water, sour or *Amla* has earth and fire in it, salty or *Lavana* has fire and water, pungent or *Katu* consists of fire and air, bitter or *Tikta* contains air and space, and, last, astringent or *Kashaya* has the air and earth elements.

In addition to the elements that the tastes are composed of, it is also beneficial to understand the impact on the body, if any of the tastes are taken in excess. The details are listed below:

Sweet: can lead to laziness, weak digestion, swelling of the glands, and such diseases as diabetes and obesity.

Sour: can cause one to feel thirsty often, and to develop teeth irritation, fever, itching, and inflammation in the body.

Salty: can increase thirst and cause skin diseases, muscle degradation, and graying of the hair.

Pungent: causes back pain, dizziness, weakness, and burning sensations in the body, affecting the reproductive organs.

Bitter: leads to joint problems, dizziness, and the degradation of the tissues.

Astringent: causes constipation and flatulence, reduces vitality and strength of the body, and causes general dryness.

What is the importance of eating with one's hands in the Vedic tradition?
According to Ayurveda, each cell in the body consists of the five natural elements, and the hands and fingers are considered to be the conduits of the same. In fact, through the thumb we experience space, the forefinger gives us the feeling of air, through the midfinger we feel the element of fire, through the ring finger we learn about the water element, and, finally, through the little finger we perceive earth. These five elements in the fingers allow the food to become digestible before it reaches the mouth, which is why eating with one's hands is customary for Indian cuisine from ancient times.

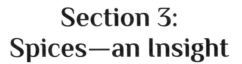

Section 3:
Spices—an Insight

Herbs and spices are an enticing addition to a dish. Spices have a dual impact—they flavor food and have healing benefits on the body. Ayurveda believes that like all living organisms, spices too have a combination of the five natural elements (earth, water, space, fire, and air).

What are the common spices and their advantages?
A glimpse into the common spices is provided below:

List of Spices

Spice	Impact
Red chili	Helps with lung congestion, boosts immunity and metabolism.
Black pepper	Treats cough, cold, and sinus issues; reduces gas; and improves digestion.
Coriander	Assists with allergies and acidity, improves digestion and appetite, and lowers blood sugar.
Cumin	Good for digestion, increases metabolism, lowers blood sugar, and promotes weight loss.
Turmeric	Reduces high cholesterol and helps with weight reduction, skin infection, and joint pain.
Mustard	Improves digestion and metabolism and helps with migraines.
Garlic	Assists with respiratory infection and cold and lowers blood pressure.
Ginger	Aids with reducing joint pain and nausea, decreases gas, and increases blood flow in the body.
Curry leaves	Makes hair strong and improves the skin condition.

It is essential to store the spices in airtight containers and keep them in a cool, dark place, to extend the spice's strength for the long term. It is not suggested to put the spices in the refrigerator, since humidity can cause the growth of bacteria or mold. If you wish to store them in the refrigerator, ensure that they have been completely vacuum-sealed. Spices are best enjoyed when they are fresh, so you can buy smaller quantities if you prefer. In order to avoid any contact with moisture, use a dry spoon while delving into the spice bowl or jar.

In India, the summer season is also the "mango" season, and in traditional households, you will find the housewives very busy making all kinds of sweet and sour mango pickles. As a child, I remember my maternal grandmother passionately seasoning the sun-dried mango pieces and helping her neighbors mix the appropriate amount of spices to make the most-delicious, lip-smacking pickles! I was always amazed at how she lovingly mixed in the right amount of salt, red chili powder, and cumin powder with her hands, without having to depend on any measuring tools.

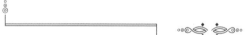

What are the favored Ayurvedic herbs?

The science of Ayurveda uses herbs as one of the treatment options for improving our physical, mental, and emotional health. A glimpse into a few of the favored Ayurvedic herbs is given below. *(Disclaimer: please do not take these without consulting an Ayurvedic doctor or Ayurvedacharya.)*:

Ashwagandha: *Ashwagandha* was first described in the *Charaka* and *Sushruta Samhitas*—the ancient Ayurvedic scriptures from India. This herb was widely used in the Middle East, India, and North Africa. It is a rejuvenating herb and can increase one's lifespan. Ashwagandha has been used for relieving physical and emotional discomfort and increasing the body's stability.

Good for: reduces stress and blood sugar levels, helps with depression, and increases muscle strength.

Brahmi: *Brahmi* is also known as *Bacopa*. It is native to India and Sri Lanka but is also grown in the southern US and Australia. This is a popular herb that is known for improving memory and concentration. It was utilized in ancient Vedic times by sages or scholars to aid them in memorizing hymns and the Vedic scriptures.[1]

Good for: lowers anxiety, prevents hair fall, rebuilds the brain tissues, improves memory and immunity.

Kutaj: *Kutaj* was first described in the *Charaka Samhita* and *Sushruta Samhita*—the ancient Ayurvedic scriptures from India. It grows in the sub-Himalayan regions. Kutaj is known to cure gastrointestinal disorders, especially diarrhea, arthritis (osteo and rheumatoid), and blood-related disorders, and boosts the overall immunity of the body. (*Note: This herb may be available only through Ayurvedic websites or practitioners in the U.S.*)

Good for: Heals stomach issues, diarrhea, kidney issues, and skin infections.

Guggul: *Guggul* can be found in Africa, the Middle East, and northern India. This herb is used for urinary and skin disorders (*Do not take if you are pregnant, breast feeding, or have severe liver or kidney disease.*)

Good for: lowers high cholesterol and weight, assists with joint pain and skin disease.

Triphala: *Triphala* originated in India as a part of Ayurvedic medicine. It is made up of the fruits of three trees that grow in India and the Middle East—Amalaki, Bhibhitaki, and Haritaki. The fruits are dried and ground into a fine powder. The Amalaki fruit, *Amla*, is Indian gooseberry, which contains high levels of vitamin C and has a cooling effect on the body. Bhibhitaki has a warming effect, and Haritaki has a rejuvenating impact.

Good for: a gentle laxative for stomach and intestines, reduces gases, removes fat, is a blood builder, and improves immunity.

Gotu Kola: this herb grows in the Himalayas and has been a part of Ayurvedic medicine from Vedic times. *Gotu kola* is from the parsley family and is an integral part both of Ayurvedic and Chinese medicine.

This herb helps with circulation of the blood and is beneficial for treating any scars on the skin. It increases the production of collagen, which helps in the process of healing.

Good for: helps with skin disease, improves blood circulation, and is good for the liver and kidneys.

Ghee: this is simply clarified butter and is known as an elixir in Ayurveda. In ancient times, ghee was hand-churned and was considered a Sattvic food that was fit to be an offering to Paramatma (Divine). This practice still continues in some Indian homes even today. Ghee is known to increase immunity, make the body and bones strong, improve the quality of skin and hair, control blood pressure, improve memory, help with insomnia, and improve one's mood.

Honey: contains a sugar that digests quickly; it is lower than sugar on the glycemic index and provides immediate energy. It is good for the eyes and skin, acts as a sedative, and assists with cough, cold, and asthma. Interestingly, honey is also known to stop hiccups.

Coriander and Cumin powders are good for digestion.
Black Pepper powder helps assimilate and better absorb
Turmeric powder in the body.

Section 4:
Fun with Spices

In my teens, my warmhearted and loving maternal grandmother taught me how to cook with spices. I have shared her recipes along with others that I enjoy making for family and friends:

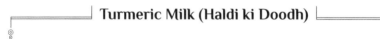

Turmeric Milk (Haldi ki Doodh)

Serves 1
Good for: all three Doshas

Ingredients:
1 cup milk (cow's or almond)
1 teaspoon organic honey
½ teaspoon turmeric powder

Method:
1. In a pot, pour the milk and add in the turmeric powder. Bring to a boil.
2. In a cup, put in the honey and pour in the boiled milk.
3. Stir and serve hot.

Potato Vegetable (Aloo ki Sabzi)

Serves 2
Good for: all three Doshas

Ingredients:
2 boiled potatoes
1 tablespoon olive oil
½ teaspoon cumin seeds
1 dry red chili
½ teaspoon red chili powder
½ teaspoon turmeric powder
¼ teaspoon dry mango powder
1 teaspoon coriander-cumin powder
½ teaspoon lemon juice (optional)
1 tablespoon finely chopped cilantro
A pinch of black pepper powder
Salt to taste

Method:
1. Chop the boiled potatoes into small pieces.
2. In a pan/wok, pour in the oil and, when it's slightly hot, add in the dry red chili and cumin seeds.
3. Once the seeds splutter for a few seconds, lower the heat and add in the chopped potatoes.
4. Add in all the spices, stir, and cook for about 5 minutes.
5. Garnish with lemon juice and chopped cilantro. Serve hot.

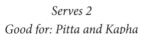

Spicy Salad

Serves 2
Good for: Pitta and Kapha

Ingredients:
1 cup chopped Chinese cabbage or spinach
½ cup grated carrots
½ cup grated beetroot
½ cup bean sprouts
¼ cup grated red radish
½ cup chopped spring onions (in thin slivers)
2 green chilis, finely chopped
½ inch fresh ginger, chopped (in thin slivers)
1 tablespoon olive oil
1 teaspoon roasted cumin seeds
½ teaspoon roasted fennel seeds
½ teaspoon red chili powder
¼ teaspoon turmeric powder
¼ teaspoon crushed mustard powder
½ teaspoon black pepper powder
½ teaspoon fresh garlic, finely chopped
¾ teaspoon organic honey
6–8 raisins
5–6 pistachios (without shells)
1 teaspoon lemon juice
Salt to taste

Method:
1. In a bowl, place the Chinese cabbage or spinach, ginger, green chilis, garlic, and grated vegetables.
2. In a blender, pour in the oil, lemon juice, red chili powder, mustard powder, salt, black pepper powder, and turmeric powder and blend to an even mixture.
3. Add the oil blend to the salad-and-vegetable mixture in the bowl.
4. Sprinkle with honey and mix well. Put in the fridge for 10–15 minutes to allow the salad to become cold.
5. Garnish with roasted cumin seeds, fennel seeds, raisins, and pistachios. Serve.

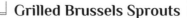

Grilled Brussels Sprouts

Serves 1
Good for: Kapha

Ingredients:
1 cup chopped brussels sprouts
1 teaspoon olive oil
½ teaspoon turmeric powder
½ teaspoon red chili powder
½ teaspoon coriander-cumin powder
¼ teaspoon ginger powder (optional)
¼ teaspoon garlic powder (optional)
¼ teaspoon black pepper powder
Salt to taste

Method:
1. In a bowl, place in the chopped brussels sprouts, add in the oil, and then add the spices. Mix well.
2. Set the oven to 370° Fahrenheit or 188° Centigrade. Spread out the mixed brussels sprouts on a baking tray and bake for 15 minutes.
3. Once grilled with a light-brown tinge, remove and serve hot.
(Note: You can substitute the brussels sprouts with broccoli or cauliflower.)

Yellow Lentils (Dal)

Serves 2
Good for: Pitta and Kapha

Ingredients:
½ cup yellow (moong) lentils
1 cup water
½ teaspoon ghee
½ teaspoon mustard seeds
½ teaspoon cumin seeds
A pinch of asafoetida
1 dry red chili
1 bay leaf
1 cardamom pod
2 cloves
½ tomato, chopped finely
1 medium onion, chopped finely
½ teaspoon crushed, fresh ginger
½ teaspoon crushed, fresh garlic
½ teaspoon turmeric powder
½ teaspoon red chili powder
½ teaspoon coriander-cumin powder
1 tablespoon finely chopped cilantro
1 teaspoon lemon juice
A pinch of black pepper powder
Salt to taste

Method:
1. In a bowl, soak the yellow (moong) lentils in water for 30 minutes, prior to cooking.
2. In a pot, boil the soaked lentils until soft. Transfer into the bowl and make into a smooth consistency with a hand mixer.
3. In the pot, heat the ghee, then add in the clove, cardamom, bay leaf, dry red chili, asafoetida, and mustard seeds. When the seeds begin to splutter, add in the cumin seeds.
4. Once the cumin seeds also splutter or become light brown, add in the onions and sauté for 5 minutes.
5. Add in the tomatoes and spices and cook for 5–10 minutes, until it becomes a paste.
6. Pour in the lentils, mix, add in the water, and cook for 10 minutes until it comes to a boil.
7. Remove, then garnish with lemon juice and the chopped cilantro. Serve hot.

Moong Dal (Yellow Lentil) Pancake

Serves 2
Good for: Pitta and Kapha

Ingredients:
1 cup yellow (moong) lentils
½ teaspoon ghee
½ teaspoon cumin seeds
½ teaspoon Eno fruit salt (*can be purchased in an Indian store*)
½ tomato, chopped finely
½ medium onion, chopped finely
¼ green pepper, chopped finely
¼ cup finely grated carrot
½ teaspoon crushed, fresh ginger
½ teaspoon crushed, fresh garlic
½ teaspoon turmeric powder
½ teaspoon red chili powder
1 tablespoon gram flour
1 tablespoon finely chopped cilantro
A pinch of black pepper powder
Salt to taste

Method:
1. In a bowl, soak the yellow (moong) lentils in water for 30 minutes. Drain and blend in a blender into a fine paste.
2. In a mixing bowl, add in the lentil paste, gram flour, vegetables, and spices. Add in the Eno fruit salt and mix well.
3. Preheat a round, flat pan and pour in the above mixture, spreading it to form a pancake shape.
4. Cook on one side for about 2–5 minutes on a low-medium flame and then flip over. The bottom side should have a light-brown color.
5. Add the ghee on the top and sides and cook until the outer crust of the pancake has a light-brown color with a crispy tinge. Ensure that the pancake is not raw in the middle.
6. Serve hot with chutney or yogurt, depending on your taste.

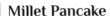
Millet Pancake

Serves 2
Good for: Kapha

Ingredients:
1 cup millet flour
½ medium onion, chopped finely
¼ cup finely grated zucchini
¼ cup finely grated carrot
¼ cup finely chopped scallions
½ teaspoon crushed, fresh ginger
½ teaspoon crushed, fresh green chilis
½ teaspoon turmeric powder
½ teaspoon red chili powder
1 tablespoon finely chopped cilantro
¾ cup water
8" squares of butter paper
2 tablespoons olive oil
A pinch of black pepper powder
Salt to taste

Method:
1. In a bowl, put in millet flour, vegetables, and spices and mix well.
2. Add in water slowly as needed to form a dough that is soft and spreadable.
3. Take a small ball of the mixture and place on the butter paper square, wet your hand, and press the ball into the shape of a pancake.
4. Heat a flat plan, place the pancake on it, add ½ teaspoon of oil, and cook until light brown. Flip and cook on the other side.
5. Serve hot with chutney or yogurt, depending on your taste.

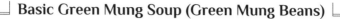

Basic Green Mung Soup (Green Mung Beans)

Serves 4
Good for: Pitta and Kapha

Ingredients:
¾ cup green mung beans
1 cup water
1 teaspoon ghee
½ teaspoon mustard seeds
½ teaspoon cumin seeds
A pinch of asafoetida
1 dry red chili
1 bay leaf
1 cardamom pod
2 cloves
¾ teaspoon crushed, fresh ginger
¾ teaspoon crushed, fresh green chilis
½ teaspoon crushed, fresh garlic
½ teaspoon turmeric powder
½ teaspoon garam masala
½ teaspoon coriander-cumin powder
1 tablespoon finely chopped cilantro
1 teaspoon lemon juice
A pinch of black pepper powder
Salt to taste

Method:
1. In a bowl, soak the green mung lentils in water for 4 hours or overnight, prior to cooking.
2. In the pot, heat the ghee, then add in the clove, cardamom, bay leaf, dry red chili, asafoetida, and mustard seeds. When the seeds begin to splutter, add in the cumin seeds.
4. Once the cumin seeds also splutter or become light brown, add in the soaked green mung beans, water, and salt and cook for 5 minutes, until the mung beans become tender, so that you can mix well to make a thick soup.
5. Add in the spices and cook for 10–12 minutes on a low-medium flame until soup is cooked and is flavorful.
6. Garnish with lemon juice and cilantro. Serve hot.

Corn and Green Pepper Rice

Serves 6
Good for: Kapha (in moderation)

Ingredients:
1 cup basmati rice (uncooked)
1.5 cup water
½ cup corn kernels
½ cup finely chopped green peppers
½ cup finely chopped onion
1 tablespoon dry or fresh coconut powder
2 tablespoons ghee
1 teaspoon cumin seeds
2 dry red chilis
1 bay leaf
1 cardamom pod
1 clove
1 piece fresh ginger (½ inch long)
2 fresh green chilis
3 cloves of fresh garlic
½ teaspoon turmeric powder
½ teaspoon garam masala
¾ teaspoon red chili powder
1 tablespoon finely chopped cilantro
A pinch of black pepper powder
Salt to taste

Method:
1. In a pot, heat the ghee. Add in the clove, cardamom, bay leaf, dry red chili, and cumin seeds.
2. Once the cumin seeds splutter or become light brown, add in the onions, corn, and green pepper and sauté for 5 minutes.
3. Take the ginger, green chilis, and garlic and blend in a blender to make a paste.
4. Add in the rice and sauté for 2 minutes. Add in the ginger–garlic–green chili paste, coconut powder, and spices and mix well.
5. Pour in the water as needed and cook the rice until tender.
6. Garnish with cilantro and serve hot.

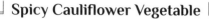

Spicy Cauliflower Vegetable

Serves 6
Good for: Pitta and Kapha

Ingredients:

1 lb. cauliflower	2 fresh green chilis
2 potatoes	6 cloves fresh garlic
1 cup peas	½ cup finely chopped cilantro
1 bay leaf	½ teaspoon turmeric powder
1 dry red chili	2 teaspoons coriander-cumin powder
¾ teaspoon mustard seeds	½ teaspoon red chili powder
¾ teaspoon cumin seeds	2 teaspoons ghee
A pinch of asafoetida	½ teaspoon garam masala
A pinch of black pepper powder	¾ cup water
2 onions, finely chopped	1 teaspoon lemon juice
2 tablespoons dry or fresh coconut powder	Salt to taste
1 inch fresh ginger	

Method:

1. Cut the vegetables into medium-sized pieces.
2. Put the cilantro (leaving aside a small amount for garnishing), ginger, green chilis, garlic, and onion in a blender and make into a paste.
3. In a pot, heat the ghee. Add in the bay leaf, the dry red chili, asafoetida, and mustard seeds. When they splutter, add in the cumin seeds.
4. Once they splutter, add in the vegetables and salt and sauté for 5 minutes.
5. Add in the paste and spices and mix well.
6. Pour in the water, cover, and cook the vegetables until tender. Stir in between so the vegetables do not stick to the pot base, which also allows the spice paste to mix in evenly.
7. Garnish with lemon juice and cilantro. Serve hot with Indian bread (roti or paratha).

Date Balls

Serves 4
Good for: Pitta

Ingredients:
1 cup pitted dates
½ teaspoon ghee
½ teaspoon cinnamon powder
¼ teaspoon ginger powder
½ teaspoon cardamom powder
¼ teaspoon red chili powder
¼ cup chopped walnuts
¼ cup chopped pistachios
¼ cup chopped cashews
3 tablespoon coconut powder or coconut flakes

Method:
1. In a bowl, put in the dates, and make them soft by putting them in the microwave for one minute or heating them on the stove by placing over a pot of water.
2. Let the dates cool for 5–10 minutes and mash into a paste.
3. Add in the spices, dried fruits, and one tablespoon coconut powder/flakes.
4. Moisten your palms with ghee, mix the date mixture, and roll into small balls.
5. Roll each ball in the remaining two tablespoons of coconut powder/flakes. Set aside to cool.
6. Put in the fridge for 60 minutes to bind more. Enjoy as a dessert or a snack.

Brown Rice Khichadi

Serves 1
Good for: Vata and Pitta

Ingredients:
¼ cup whole moong dal
¼ cup brown basmati rice
⅛ tablespoon ghee
¼ teaspoon black peppercorns
¼ teaspoon cumin seeds
¼ teaspoon turmeric powder
1 cup of boiling water
A pinch of salt
A pinch of asafoetida

Method:
1. Soak the moong dal in 1 cup of water at room temperature for 2 hours and drain. Wash the rice and dal until the water becomes clear.
2. In a large, deep pot, heat the ghee. Add in asafoetida, peppercorns, and cumin seeds and sauté.
3. Add the rice and dal. Sauté over low heat for 3 minutes.
4. Add the boiling water, salt, and turmeric powder.
5. Cover and simmer over a low heat for 1 hour, stirring to prevent it from burning. Serve hot.

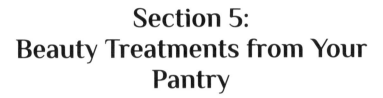

Section 5:
Beauty Treatments from Your Pantry

Our pantry and kitchen at home provide us with some wonderful ingredients that can help us maintain our beauty regimen without having to resort to store-bought products, if so preferred.

What are the accessible natural beauty products in your kitchen?
The list below is a glimpse into some of these magical items:

Honey: a natural moisturizer and hair conditioner.

Fenugreek: helps clean the hair follicles and scalp. It is best mixed with a base oil such as coconut oil and massaged into the scalp.

Shikakai: acts as a hair conditioner and removes dandruff.

Potato or cucumber slices: helps remove dark circles around the eyes. Place freshly cut slices on your eyelids for a few minutes once your eyes are closed.

Multani Mitti **or Fuller's earth**: for tightening and rejuvenating skin. Mix with water or rosewater and a pinch of turmeric powder and apply to the face and neck. Wash off with warm water once dry.

Rice powder: acts as an exfoliator, giving skin a new radiance.

Neem oil: can be used on minor inflammation such as pimples, especially during the summer season, since it has a cooling effect.

Aloe vera: makes the skin supple and soft. You can apply externally on the skin or consume it in a healthful beverage.

Rosewater: is a wonderful toner.

Sandalwood powder: good for acne, blemishes, and wrinkles. Mix with water or rosewater and apply to the face and neck. Wash off with luke-warm water once dry.

Coconut oil: stimulates hair growth and shine. Massage into the hair and scalp, keep on for about an hour, and wash off with warm water. In addition, swishing coconut oil in the mouth is good for oral hygiene. (*Suggestion: Do not discard in your basin but in the trash can, to prevent the oil from clogging the pipes.*)

Dry-brush your body with a natural-bristle brush to tone the skin and reduce cellulite. It is best done in a circular motion and moving upward toward the heart.

Lastly, do a self-massage with base oils such as coconut or sesame oil, especially in the winter season just before you shower. (*Disclaimer: It is best to do a small test patch first to ensure that the oil does not cause any inflammation or rash on the skin.*) In Ayurveda, it is believed that anything that is put on the skin is absorbed in the body within 45 minutes.

There are certain suggestions for skin care for the three *Dosha* types:

Vata: Vata individuals tend to have dry skin and could age faster due to the elements of air and space. In order to counter this, it is best to use skin care products that are nurturing and hydrating. It is recommended to drink lukewarm water throughout the day to stay hydrated. A morning self-massage with sesame or avocado oil is suggested, and facial skin can be moisturized with natural products such as sesame oil, aloe vera, and vegetable glycerin.

Pitta: Pitta individuals tend to have oily and sensitive skin, so cooling and nurturing products are recommended. It is best to stay away from chemical-based cosmetics since they can contribute to breakouts or acne. A self-massage with cooling oils such as jojoba or grapeseed oil is best. The use of gentle moisturizers containing honey, aloe vera, and grapeseed oil is suggested. It is good to take precautionary measures to protect Pittas' sensitive skin from the direct rays of the sun.

Kapha: Kapha individuals have skin that tends to be more thick and oily, so cleansing both externally and internally is required. Externally, you can use gentle scrubs such as chickpea or barley flour to cleanse the skin, while internally, doing a regular detox is helpful. A self-massage every morning with grapeseed or corn oil, along with regular exercise, is advantageous for improving circulation.

Section 6:
Spiritual Concepts

What do spirituality, compassion, and empathy mean?

Spirituality is when one believes that there is something greater than the material human existence. One believes in spirit or in a higher power that is part of the Divine and the Cosmic Universe. Each living being contains in them a soul or *Atma* that is a part of Higher Consciousness or the Divine or Paramatma, which is also known as your guiding light or I AM. This is what is termed as *sentient*.

Empathy is the emotional kindness that we can extend to others with awareness to really understand how the other feels. It is the basis of emotional intelligence, without which we cannot truly listen to another human being and their troubles.

Compassion is a feeling of sympathy that we feel for others that propels us to take action. This feeling arises when we see someone in pain or trouble, and we feel a need internally to send them healing light and love, whether they are in proximity or at a distance. Compassion comes from the heart and can be felt toward all living beings.

A feeling of compassion arises when we become more aware of our own selves and others, and this happens when we slow down and live in the present moment. Another criterion (which I have explained in more detail below) is to develop a mindset of *nonjudgment*.

It is often easier to have compassion for our family and friends, especially when they approach us with their problems. However, most people in general do not understand the notion of self-compassion. It is similar to the instruction that we receive when we board a flight. The flight attendant advises us to secure our own oxygen masks before taking this protective action for our family or companions travelling with us. In the same way, if your own energy is depleted, how can you effectively extend compassion and understanding to another?

We often use critical words toward ourselves, which is the opposite of compassion, and this in turn makes us internally unhappy. It is when we recognize our own suffering and take loving action to help ourselves that we begin to feel tranquil and untroubled. Once we achieve this for ourselves, we become motivated to extend this sympathetic love and care to others.

Compassion toward family and friends is easier than extending nondiscriminatory care toward people who we don't really know—in short, humanity at large. This is where we all must try to recognize that we are part of the same humanity; we all are one and come from the same source. This will motivate us to extend the highest healing power there is—love!

I expect to pass through life but once. If, therefore, there be any kindness I can show, or any good thing I can do to any fellow being, let me do it now and not defer or neglect it, as I shall not pass this way again.

—William Penn[1]

What is Seva?

Seva in Sanskrit means *selfless service*. It is a heart-centered, compassionate desire to improve and uplift the life condition of those around you. This can be done in many ways in our day-to-day lives, for example:

Volunteering: volunteer your time and skills in imparting knowledge to others who need it. It could be as a mentor to a someone who is trying to start their career or as easy as reading a book to a child in a children's home.

Respect: through small gestures: give respect to the elderly or a pregnant woman by giving up your seat in the bus or subway. If you see an elderly couple trying to hail a cab on the street, stop and help them do this. They will really appreciate your *Seva*.

Payment: if you are at the coffee shop or a restaurant, offer to pay for someone. The idea is not to judge the other person's circumstance, but just to give selflessly because it creates a circle of good karma.

Smiling: this is one of easiest ways to serve. Smile when you enter a room or when you meet someone. You have no idea how the other person's day has been, and your smile might be the only ray of hope for them in that moment.

Generosity: be generous to those who are needy. You can be walking on the street, and if you see a homeless person, give them money or buy them food, and while doing so, ask Paramatma to bless them. If you can't give them monetary help, a quick prayer for their well-being is a wonderful *selfless service*.

The above also creates beautiful good karma for yourself, but the true essence of *Seva* is to do the action without any expectation of return from the recipient or from Paramatma. After all, we are all connected, and through *Seva* you are doing your dharma as a sentient being.

What is intuition?

Intuition is what we refer to as internal knowing and getting answers from our sixth sense or I AM. These messages are provided physically, mentally, or emotionally and can be presented through feelings, signs, and messages as a revelation. Pay attention to your mind and body—if you feel a strong sense of comfort when faced with a situation or person, know that you are on the right track, but if there is an inner dread or even slight discomfort, then your intuition is guiding you to be careful.

In addition to the messages we get through intuition, the Cosmic Universe also provides us answers through symbols or signs. For example, pigeons or doves represent love and sacrifice, and the numbers 11:11 may symbolize the opening of a spiritual portal.

What does it mean to forgive and let go?

In our human existence when someone hurts us, we feel offended, but it would be useful to understand that what really gets affected is our ego. This pain remains in our mind and memory, and we often hang on to it with a feeling of wanting to get back at them or hurt them. In our path toward spirituality, we learn that the heart or love is greater than the mind and ego; therefore, it is preferable to deal with the suffering, forgive the other person (who caused you the pain), and let go. This does not mean that we are allowing the other person to get off the hook, especially if what they did is unacceptable, but giving ourselves permission to be free from pain—in short, emotional freedom.

If we do not forgive, and continue to hold on to the pain, anger, negative thoughts, and hurt, we cause ourselves more pain. In true forgiveness we are able to transcend our ego and release ourselves of the pain that we are holding on to by letting go. To illustrate, let go of a ball that you are holding in your hand, and really feel the space. Similarly, after you forgive and let go, you have intentionally created space in your heart along with peace of mind, and the painful scenario no longer has any intensity or hold on you. You become emotionally and spiritually free.

Why is nonjudgment related to spiritual growth?

It is crucial to realize that when we judge another, we are not accepting them as they are. We are assigning them a label, and by doing that we are restricting our perception of them. If we feel entitled to place a label on someone, or judge them, we must question that in doing so, are we stuck in our ego? The answer will mostly be in the affirmative.

It does not make this behavior right or make us superior in any capacity. Additionally, it also limits our own thinking, since we cannot see the different dimensions of the person or situation. Spiritually, it even hinders our own ascension. Sometimes, when we judge others it is because we are dealing with some insecurity, and through the judgment we project this insecurity on the other. This is detrimental to us in the long term since we avoid healing ourselves. If we can be observant of our thoughts and actions on a regular basis, it will be the first step to spiritual freedom, and freedom from the incessant need to judge others.

The second method is through meditation. Meditation allows us to calm down and reduce our stress levels. Over time, we are no longer in a negative state ourselves, and therefore we don't resort to a negative perception of others as a natural reaction. As we raise our own vibration, our perception of our own self and others transforms.

In nonjudgment, you allow yourself to be more open to receiving and giving love, which results in personal freedom and happiness. You accept people and situations as they are, flowing with the *Universe,* and in doing so, you receive that wonderful energy back too. Spiritually, you become stronger and avoid being pulled into any nonconstructive drama as you begin to recognize the I AM (Divine) in others.

What is Karma and how does this affect us in our lives?

Karma literally means *action*, which is an important concept in Vedic spirituality. Every action and intention will have a related reaction or effect. If you have an honest and good thought, intention, emotion, or action toward another, with an intention to offer help, support, and kindness, it will result in good karma. However, if you have a mean or negative intention, thought, or action toward another, then you will attract negative or bad karma to yourself. Take for example a person who is jealous and takes a manipulative stance or action toward another—in the long run, he/she will never see a positive result for this stance.

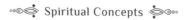

Illustration

You are interested in someone, and they chose to marry another person. Understandably you feel heartbroken. However, if you still try to connect with this person in an intimate way, knowing that they are committed to someone else, then you have created negative karma for yourself. It is more about respecting their decision, overcoming your own emotional attachment toward them, and letting go.

If, however, you maintain integrity in your interactions and relationships, then the positive fruits of that will also come back to you as rewards. In the Vedic context, karma extends not only to the current but also to past and future lives, in what is known as the *Karmic cycle*. Until you learn the lesson that the Universe is trying to teach you for your spiritual growth, you will be tied to that karmic cycle, irrespective of whether the inception of that was in this or a previous lifetime. It is therefore advised to have high integrity in your life.

You reap what you sow . . .

Section 7:
Spiritual Healing

What is healing?

Healing is a process where we use different techniques to become healthy on a physical, psychological, emotional, and spiritual level.

What is gratitude?

Gratitude means thanks or appreciation. It is a way of recognizing what the *Universe* or someone has done for you. In giving thanks, you raise yourself to a higher, more positive vibration, which in turn opens you up to more good news and opportunities. This improves your health and well-being and strengthens your ability to handle problems or adversity. In addition, show appreciation to your family and friends when they do something nice for you. Everyone likes to feel appreciated, so say *thank you* when someone does a kind deed for you and takes care of you, even if it is your family member. Smiling is another way to convey a positive emotion and respect.

What is meditation?

The essence of meditation is to go beyond the mind, or what is known as *no mind*. Anything can be meditation as long as we are in total awareness in the present moment, to the extent where we are no longer even conscious of the passing of time.

Meditation allows us to connect with Paramatma and attain a state of calm and equilibrium or *Stithpragya*, where we are not affected by external situations or difficulties. Meditation done over a period of time will allow our internal light to become steady and guide us, removing negative emotions such as anxiety, worry, fear, and anger.

It is advised to make it a daily practice, preferably in the morning—find a corner in your home that can be your meditation alcove; sit cross-legged, with your back straight, palms resting on your lap, close your eyes and sit in quiet contemplation. If you can find a corner where you are facing the morning sun, you begin to feel each ray of the sun filling you with positive energy and brilliance, vibrancy, and good health.

It is best not to try to force yourself to stop your thoughts during meditation, but to relax and allow your thoughts to just pass through. In this process, you become the observer of what is going on in your mind without any judgment, and you develop an awareness of the Cosmic Universe. Over time, the random thoughts in your mind will slow down and disappear, allowing you to listen to the guidance from the Universe.

The corner of your home where you practice daily is your *meditation sanctuary*, which you can arrange in a manner that is truly personal to you. You can adorn it with flowers, crystals, candlelights, photos, statues, motivating thoughts, spiritual affirmations, and beads. As you connect to this divine personal space, it will become a focal point for you, and you will find over time that you are intrinsically drawn to it each morning. It becomes your personal go-to space for love and light.

A regular practice of meditation provides the following benefits:
- reduces stress and pain
- increases a positive outlook in life
- increases attention span and memory
- improves sleep
- helps deal with addictions
- allows you to think in a calm and peaceful manner before taking decisions
- provides a higher vibration and encourages spirituality

The technique of how to do meditation has been described above. However, anything done with complete immersion and with full awareness can be described as meditation—if you are having a cup of morning tea at the start of your day, for example, be focused on that cup of tea and each sip of tea that you are taking—the smell, taste, and impact. You are completely in the moment, fully absorbed, with no distractions in your mind. It is in being in total enjoyment of drinking your cup of morning tea that it becomes a sublime experience, which, in short, is meditation.

How do crystals help elevate positive, healing energies?

In the ancient Vedic times, the holistic approach (mind-body-spirit) extended to the use of crystals and gemstones, since they believed that crystals had healing energies to balance the mental, physical, emotional, and astral bodies. In particular, gemstones were used to fix certain physical issues and to get relief from emotional blockages.

Our physical bodies have an energy vibration around it, which is referred to as an *aura*. The crystals that are placed on the body cause a surge of energy into the body, thereby transmitting their healing power to bring about a realignment to our overall energy vibration or aura.

A few of the common crystals are:

- **Amethyst:** helps with emotionality and increases peace, contentment, intuition, insight, and spirituality
- **Aquamarine:** protects during major life changes, removes stress and anxiety, and raises Higher Consciousness
- **Aventurine:** brings about good luck, manifestation, and confidence
- **Black tourmaline:** increases grounding, security, and removal of negative energy
- **Citrine:** raises confidence, positivity, joy, and overall lightness
- **Clear quartz:** important for clarity, illumination, and manifestation
- **Diamond:** rejuvenates, raises spirituality, and brings prosperity
- **Garnet:** removes blockages, increases passion, and energizes
- **Jade:** for wisdom, good luck, and success
- **Lapis lazuli:** a sacred stone that gives strength to the mind, body, and spirit
- **Onyx:** for calmness, protection, and balance
- **Pearl:** promotes vitality and strength
- **Rose quartz:** for unconditional love, peace, compassion, and forgiveness
- **Ruby:** for concentration and mental power
- **Topaz:** relieves fear and increases passion
- **Turquoise:** increases wisdom, protection, and high vibrations

How can essential oils help us?

Essential oils are extracted from herbs, plants, flowers, fruits, and whole spices. Each essential oil has healing benefits and should be mixed with base oils such as almond, coconut, and olive oil before application. These essential oils are obtained from the fresh herbs/flowers.

The specific effects of the popular essential oils are:

- **Lavender:** calming and relaxing
- **Peppermint:** rejuvenating and uplifting
- **Tea tree:** cleansing and purifying
- **Rosemary:** cleansing and purifying
- **Frankincense:** calming and grounding
- **Rose:** soothing and hydrating
- **Sandalwood:** calming and enhances spirituality

What is color therapy?

Color therapy is when we use the vibrations of colors for healing, and is similar to the concept of using crystals for their energy or vibration. Color therapy can be through the color in a room, clothes, gems that we wear, and food that we eat. A color viewed by the eyes is assimilated by the brain, is absorbed by the nervous system, and causes cellular and hormonal changes.

Each color contains its own unique energy, which influences a specific organ in the body, and all seven colors in the spectrum are essential to maintain the balance for our well-being: red, orange, yellow, green, blue, indigo, and violet. Gems contain the seven colors as in light, and this energy is absorbed by our inner or subtle body to bring about healing. To be specific, colors have a direct impact in accordance with one's *Dosha*:

- *Vata*: yellow, red, orange, green
- *Pitta*: green, blue, purple, indigo
- *Kapha*: yellow, red, orange, purple, indigo

How can we learn from nature and transform?

There are different examples in nature from which we can deeply understand the process of transformation. If you look at a phoenix, it is a magnificent bird that dies with a burst of flames and is then reborn from the ashes with a new body. What a beautiful concept! This teaches us that at any time, we can literally transform our old ways of being to become a stronger, new version of ourselves.

If you look at a lotus pond, the flower petals bloom so beautifully, yet the water it grows in is muddy and murky. Similarly, even if we face dire circumstances or an unexpected negative situation, we can learn to have faith, stand in our own power, and not lean toward negativity. Instead, remain internally strong and positive, sure of the fact that we can rise above the difficulties, which are a blip in the spectrum of a lifetime.

In the case of a relationship issue where we feel that we have been treated badly or unfairly, it is natural to be upset or angry. However, realize that in holding on to anger and not forgiving the other person, we are keeping ourselves in the negative quagmire, causing more injury to ourselves. Instead of reacting, it is more useful to develop insight and detachment as a means to handle the situation and thereby raise our own personal vibration toward understanding the other person, including ourselves. It is not always easy to do and requires much courage and inner resolve to come into emotional balance and release. Therein lies our true power for transformation and growth.

What is spiritual empowerment?

In our daily lives, it is not uncommon at times to experience a sense of meaninglessness toward the larger world out there, or with the bigger picture of our own lives. At such points, we may be unable to endure our own disconnection from others and the world at large. This causes despair and we slip into our personal addictive states—whether that is drinking or having a shopping addiction.

This disconnection occurs because we have not looked inward and tapped into our I AM, which is our guiding light. It is when we are spiritually tuned in that we can gain the capacity to plug into a deeper, more secure connection that provides us with inner strength and resilience to face what we perceive to be insurmountable issues, both personally and in the wider world.

Spiritual empowerment is the key that leads us toward inner growth and wholeness. It is connecting with something that is greater than ourselves, which in turn allows us to better care for ourselves and other living beings. Spiritual empowerment is about inner awareness where you can freely examine your beliefs and identity and tap into the mind-body-spirit connection. It is a gradual process that allows you to uncover your inherent desires and passions and to connect with your true self and the divine within you.

During the discovery process, it is not uncommon to ask yourself questions such as:
- Am I truly happy and fulfilled?
- What makes me feel dissatisfied or unhappy? What do I really value?
- Am I holding on to any negative notions?
- How do I contribute to the world?
- How can I improve myself and be a better person today?

During the process of spiritual empowerment, one of the most important facets is to consciously move your mind away from the past and the future—be fully immersed in the present moment. In doing this you will increase your awareness and tap into the unlimited source energy that will guide your growth and transformation process.

Another facet is to learn to love your true self (not your ego), but from understanding who you really are. It is essential to learn self-love by cultivating a relationship with yourself. It is only when you love your own company, and respect your own approval, that you will find yourself happily disassociating from the external approval from others, which had become a poor habit in the past. This pulls you out from being needy, where others' acceptance, love, and viewpoints determined your self-worth.

In addition, as you change you send love and good vibes to others and allow others to be themselves without judgment. In short, spiritual empowerment at its core is learning to love who you really are, and when you love yourself without judgment, you are motivated to extend that nondiscriminatory, open-minded love and compassion to others.

This helps free you from negative thought patterns that control your mind. It is when you arrange your thoughts, emotions, and energy in a positive direction and retrain your focus that you will allow the Universe to support you to achieve what you want. However, this manifestation power becomes stronger when you consider others' welfare too. You become empowered when you become conscious and nonfluctuating and have complete faith in Higher Consciousness.

Every day presents a new opportunity and, with this, abiding faith. The manifestation process comes into play so long as you are clear about what you want and do not allow any negative thoughts to enter, even during trying times. This can be done by consciously moving yourself from the external world to your inner self or I AM. This bestows inner peace, calm, and fulfillment as you take the time to listen to the guidance that your I AM continues to provide to you as a precious gift. You become a cocreator with the Universe. This is the true meaning of spiritual empowerment.

You have within you unlimited power from the Universe that has been granted to you through your I AM. It is here where you will find your true friend, lover, and the source of ever-flowing inspiration to form the most beautiful, powerful relationship with yourself, leading to beauty, joy, and the ability to manifest the new vision for your life proactively as a cocreator.

Section 8:
Vedic Healing

Shaantih Mantra / Prayer for Peace
Om Poornam-adah Poornam-idah Poorna-aat Poornam-udachyate
Om Poorna-asya Poornam-aadaaya Poornam-evaavashishsyate
Om Shaantih Shaantih Shaantih
—Shukla Yajur Veda[1]

Meaning:
Om! That Brahman is infinite, and this Universe is infinite.
The infinite proceeds from the infinite,
Then taking the infinitude of the infinite (Universe),
It remains as the infinite (Brahman) alone.
Om! Let there be peace in me.
Let there be peace in my environment.
Let there be peace in the forces that act on me.[1]

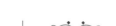
Shaantih Mantra / Universal Prayer for Peace

Om Dyauh Shaantir-Antarikssam Shaantih
Prthivii Shaantir-Aapah Shaantir-Ossadhayah Shaantih
Vanaspatayah Shaantir-Vishve-Devaah Shaantir-Brahma Shaantih
Sarvam Shaantih Shaantireva Shaantih Saa Maa Shaantir-Edhi
Om Shaantih Shaantih Shaantih

—Shukla Yajur Veda (36:17) [2]

Meaning:
May peace radiate there in the whole sky as well as in the vast
ethereal space everywhere.
May peace reign all over this earth, in water, and in all herbs,
trees, and creepers.
May peace flow over the whole universe.
May peace be in the Supreme Being Brahman.
And may there always exist in all peace and peace alone.
Om peace, peace and peace to us and all beings! [2]

What are the Vedas?

The Vedas are ancient scriptures that form the basis of Hinduism, which is also referred to as *Sanatan Dharma* (Eternal Law of Life). The origins of the Vedas have been attributed to the Indo-Aryans (though there is no concrete proof of this). One belief is that it was imparted to sages and scholars directly from God and was then passed on from generation to generation by word of mouth in Vedic Sanskrit since the second millennium BCE.

It is believed that Sage Vyasa compiled this knowledge into four collections or *Samhitas*; namely:

Rig Veda: is a compilation of more than 1,028 hymns that are organized in verse format, of which some are still recited during auspicious events such as prayer sessions *(pujas)* or at a Hindu wedding. It is the oldest known Vedic Sanskrit text in the world and was probably composed around 1700–1100 BCE.

Yajur Veda: is a collection of prose mantras focused on worship or rituals and was probably created around 1200–800 BCE. The Aryans did not always worship gods and goddesses as sculptural forms (as is commonly done in India today); rather, they cited sacred verses or mantras while making offerings in a *yajna* or holy fire.

Sama Veda: is a collection of melodies and chants that became the basis for the established tradition of music and dance. It also contains the *Chandogya* and *Kena Upanishad*, which influenced the Vedanta school of Hindu philosophy. The *Sama Veda* is believed to have been composed around 1200–1000 BCE.

Atharva Veda: contains knowledge about the procedures of life along with the rituals for marriage and funerals. It is also known as the Veda of magical formulas as it is said to have the formulas for the nature-derived potions of medicine. The Atharva Veda was composed around 1200–1100 BCE.

The Vedas teach us about the nature of the Divine and imparts knowledge about the varied aspects of life. Dharma or the essential nature states that man can be distinguished from other living beings by our potential capacity to become *divine* or *enlightened* and voluntarily embark on the spiritual path.

On the question of *how*, the Vedas state that the truth is, that Higher Consciousness or divinity is already within us as the I AM, and that we only have to discover it, connect with it, and this Supreme power will sustain us throughout life. Each person has been given the right to follow his Dharma with truth and integrity for the benefit of the whole society, community, and all living beings on earth.

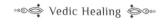
Dwavimou purushou loke,
Ksharakshara eva cha,
Kshara savani bhoothani,
Kootastho aakshara eva cha.[3]

Meaning:
Two type of men exist,
The fallible and infallible,
All living things are fallible,
And infallible among them are those,
Who are merged with the principle of God.
                    —*15–16, Tri Sloki Gita*[3]

Uthamam purushasthwanya,
Paramathmethyudahyatha,
Yo loka trayamavisya,
Bibhartha vyaya Iswara.[3]

Meaning:
But greatest among those is another,
Supreme Self, who is said to be,
That lord who is spread all over,
And maintains the three parts of the Universe.
                    —*15–17, Tri Sloki Gita*[3]

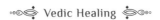

Yasmath kshara matheetho Aham,
Aksharathapi chothama,
Atho asmo loke Vede cha,
Praditha purushothama.[3]

Meaning:
Because I am beyond the fallible one,
And greatest among the infallible ones,
The world and the books of Vedas,
Call me as the most supreme personality.

—*15–18, Tri Sloki Gita*[3]

How did existence come into being according to the Vedas and Ayurveda?
According to the Vedic texts, prior to the manifestation of the Universe, there was Brahman (the absolute nonmanifested state), which comprises:

Purusha **or pure consciousness***:* which has no form and no color and is
considered to be male energy as passive witness to creation.

Prakruti **or creative will***:* which has color, form, and attributes in the field
of activity and is considered to be female power.

It is in the interplay of *Purusha and Prakruti* that the nonmaterial manifests into material expression. The conduit between the two is *Prana*, or life force, which underlies all concrete actualization. It is through the vibration of this *universal cosmic power* that the three *Gunas* or qualities—*Sattva, Rajas, and Tamas*—are created. It is specifically through the movement of these three qualities that discernible existence comes into being.

The source of all existence is the *universal cosmic power* or *consciousness* that gets manifested as *male* and *female* energy.

What is the So Ham breathing method?

This method consists of the two words *Sah* (that) *Aham* (I am). The So Ham Mantra means *I AM THAT*—the *Atma* or soul in each individual is a part of Higher Consciousness or Paramatma. In order to chant this mantra correctly, chant *so* on every breath in and *ham* on every breath out.

What is the meaning of Namaste?

Namaste is a common greeting in India. It is done by joining your palms together and bowing your head to another as a form of respect while addressing them. The recipient also responds in a similar manner. In essence, it means *I bow to you*; however, here it is important to understand that you are bowing to the Higher Consciousness or I AM or the Divine within the other person (his soul), and not his ego. It is another way of saying *I recognize the Divine in you just like I recognize the Divine in me, and I bow respectfully.*

What does Om stand for?

Om is related to the Universe or cosmos or Higher Consciousness. In the Vedic texts, Om refers to the cosmic sound and affirmation in the Divine. The sound of Om is the sound of the soul. Om is also a tool in meditation that empowers us to find the universal energy or I AM within us. Om can also be pronounced as *Aum* and covers the past, present, and future, representing the functions of creation, preservation, and transformation in a living being.

What is Karma Yoga?

This is the path of action and intention, where selfless service is known as *Nishkarma* Yoga. In this form of service, we are encouraged to act not from selfish desires but for the betterment of all. Service done with sincerity for others without any concern for return or gain is the best form of Karma Yoga. In doing this, dedicate each action to the *Supreme* as if you are serving Paramatma without any concern for the outcome. Consider this to be your duty or dharma.

The essence is in being focused yet detached and performing actions with joy and abandon. You must truly enjoy the work or service that is being done. This, in turn, will allow you to get immersed in it and be completely in the present moment.

What are Karmic ties?

In Vedic philosophy, there is a concept of *reincarnation* where the soul or nonmaterial *Self* takes a new life after the death of the physical body. *Karmic ties* are those ties that bind us to our karma both in the present and past lives.

Have you ever wondered why we meet only certain people in our life even though there are about 7.8 billion people on this planet?

We meet those karmic ties in order to finish a karmic cycle, which can also be called *unfinished business*, or to fulfill what was not fulfilled and thereby get a push forward in our spiritual growth through such an interaction. We don't meet people by coincidence; they are meant to cross our path for a reason. These karmic ties either bring us blessings or lessons (maybe through conflicts), but the truth is that if it is a lesson, until we learn it we will keep attracting it through others. Every experience is meant to teach us something.

The best approach is to therefore be observant and mindful and take appropriate action, since we are cocreators with the Universe through our karma—every action or thought has a related effect. There is nothing to fear while going through any intense karmic cycles, if you can remember at the time that these are for your spiritual ascension.

What is *Vaastu*?

Vaastu Shastra is an ancient science that gives guidance on the architecture and interior of the home to bring harmony and optimistic energy to the living space. Vaastu shastra originates in the *Atharva Veda*, and Lord Vasthoshpathe is the god of this ancient science who is known to protect homes. According to the principles of Vaastu, not only is the layout of the living space important, but also the entrance to the home, which is considered to be the entryway for energy.

In order to allow soothing energy to enter the home, the main entry door should face the north, east, or northeast in such a way that when one steps out of the door, one faces the east or northeast. The main entry door should be lit and should open in a clockwise manner. It is suggested that the door not be painted black, since this color is considered to be inauspicious.

A wonderful addition in a home is a meditation room or corner for spiritual growth. In the guidance provided by Vaastu, facing the sun in the east enhances high vibrational energy. The color scheme of rooms for personal use, like the meditation room, should be green or beige, since neutral colors enhance harmony and lightness.

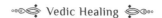

Vaastu Mantra

Vasthoshpathe,
Shagmaya samsada they sakshimahi
Ranvaya gathumathya
Pathe kshema utha yoge varam no,
Yuyam patha swasthibhi sadaa na.[4]

Meaning:
O guardian of the dwelling,
May we possess a happy home,
Which is delightful and great.
Protect our desires in peace and in action,
And, O gods, look after this house.[4]

Sraddha-Virya-Smrti-Samadhi-Prajna-Purvakah-Itaresam[5]

Meaning:
Those who follow the path of prescribed efforts and adopt the means
of reverential faith, energy, repeated recollection, concentration, and
real knowledge thus attain Samadhi.
—Patanjali Yoga Sutra (chapter 1, sutra 20).[5]

What is *Virya*?

Virya, in accordance with Patanjali's Yoga Sutra, is the *indomitable will* that is crucial for attaining *Samadhi* (contemplation). It is the will of the yogi or student to remain on the path to enlightenment and continue with the journey to Higher Consciousness. The other techniques that are crucial are unconditional faith, and belief, or *Shraddha*; memory, or *Smriti*; deep absorption of meditation, or *Samadhi*; and discernment or *Prajna*.

Faith leads to the buildup of the indomitable will, which increases one's concentration and leads to the attainment of knowledge and discernment.

What is Bhakti Yoga (chanting)?

Bhakti Yoga in the Vedas means service through love and devotion. In Bhakti Yoga, we use prayer, chanting, hymns, reading of the scriptures, and rituals to express our devotion to Paramatma with sincerity, complete faith, and a feeling of surrender. *Smaran*, or repetitive chanting of mantras, can:

- reduce stress and raise hopeful vibrations
- benefit your nervous system
- encourage spiritual development
- improve your listening skills, compassion, and love for others

One of the most powerful mantras is the universal prayer, or the *Gayatri Mantra*:

Om bhūr bhuvaḥ svaḥ
tát savitúr váreṇ(i)yaṃ
bhárgo devásya dhīmahi
dhíyo yó naḥ prachodayat

Translation:

We meditate on that most adored Supreme Lord, the creator, whose effulgence (divine light) illumines all realms (physical, mental, and spiritual). May this divine light illumine our intellect.

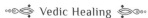

Another powerful Vedic Mantra is:

Om Nama Shivaya

Meaning:
Om: Universal Cosmic Vibration
Na: the sound of *Prithvi*, or the earth
Ma: the sound of *Jala*, or water
Shi: energies of *Agni*, or fire
Va: energies of *Vayu,* or air
Ya: energies of *Antariksha*, or space

One of the most beautiful mantras that can awaken your inner loving energy is:

Hare Krishna Hare Krishna
Krishna Krishna Hare Hare
Hare Rama Hare Rama
Rama Rama Hare Hare

This is a predominant mantra in worship of the benevolent Lord Krishna and Lord Rama, both being the incarnations of the Supreme God Vishnu and referred to in this mantra as Hare. This is also known as the *Maha Mantra* or great mantra. It is through the recitation of this mantra that a deep search for divine love is stirred, along with an awakening of consciousness.

The impact of this mantra goes beyond the mental and intellectual body to the core of one's being (heart). Love is, after all, the most powerful force in the Universe that holds everything together.

Love alone is capable of uniting living beings in such a way as to complete and fulfill them, for it alone takes them and joins them by what is deepest in themselves.

—*Pierre Teilhard de Chardin*[6]

Another aspect of Bhakti Yoga is singing *bhajans* or hymns that are in praise of the Divine and are devotional in nature. Sound energy through the singing of bhajans is therapeutic for the mind and heart (emotions). Similar to meditation, this form of Yoga can remove you from the ties of time and space and move you into the orbit of love and worship for the Divine. If the bhajan is sung from the heart center with joy and exhilaration, it will be more effective in forming that internal connection to Higher Consciousness.

Lastly, the recitation of the scriptures and rituals can go hand in hand in worship of the Divine—the choice to perform this is subjective.

This discipline of Yoga consists of eight aspects that when followed bring about a union between mind, body, and soul. In short, the word "Yoga" means *union*. These eight aspects or steps bring you closer to the connection with your Higher Self or I AM:

- *Yama*: universal cosmic vibration
- *Niyama*: individual laws of attitude that we adopt for ourselves
- *Asana*: physical Yoga practice and postures
- *Pranayama*: breath control techniques
- *Pratyhara*: control of one's senses
- *Dharana*: concentration or awareness
- *Dhyana*: meditation
- *Samadhi*: union with the Divine

What is *Yama*?

Yama is basically a code of universal morality that covers:

- ***Ahimsa***: nonviolence and compassion toward other living beings
- ***Satya***: truthfulness and honesty
- ***Pratyhara***: control of one's senses
- ***Asteya***: not taking anything that does not belong to you or that is given freely to you
- ***Brahmacharya***: sense control and behavior that is motivated toward the Absolute Truth or I AM
- ***Aparigraha***: to avoid taking advantage of a situation or without exploiting or hurting another

What is *Niyama*?

Niyama is a personal code of life and living. It is very individualistic in nature, and each person is allowed to make his own karmic choices in following these *niyamas* or rules. These niyamas include:

- ***Sauch*** or **cleanliness/purity**: This covers both external cleanliness of the body and inner purity of the mind and internal organs. External cleanliness can be through physical Yoga to remove any buildup of toxins. Inner purity of the mind is through having more productive, uplifting thoughts and ideas.
- ***Santosha*** or **contentment**: This means being content or happy with what we have in our lives and being grateful for the same, instead of clamoring unhappily about all that we don't have.
- ***Tapas*** or **discipline**: This involves *Tapas* in body and mind. Discipline in the body relates to nutrition and lifestyle. Tapas in the mind is to be dedicated to discovery of the Divine or being committed to the journey to our I AM.
- ***Svadhyaya*** or **self-study**: Being self-aware in all our activities and removing any self-destructive behavior or tendencies that are detrimental to our growth and progress.

What is *Pratyhara*?

Pratyhara means withdrawal of the senses and starts with focusing on our inner selves and letting go of our attachment to the outer world, or those things that constantly feed our senses. If this is not done, we will be distracted from the journey to our I AM or the path of *self-realization*. If we cannot control our senses, we will continually become a slave to external stimuli or situations that can destroy our inner peace and balance. It is in bringing our senses into balance rather than becoming a slave to them.

Take the example of a foodie—this is someone who is constantly drawn to good foods and lavish meals, because the sense of taste is like an addiction. However, when a person learns to eat mindfully and what is good for health, it will result in physical and emotional equilibrium.

What is *Pranayama* or breath control?

Pranayama is the process of centering your *Prana* or life force. It comprises breath control techniques such as alternate-nostril breathing, or *Nadi Shodhana*; breath of fire, or *Kapalbhati*; and victory breath, or *Ujjayi*, to name a few.

Pranayama does the following:
- allows for energy to flow freely and improves breathing in general
- lowers stress and pacifies the mind
- increases self-awareness and mindfulness
- reduces high blood pressure and helps with addictions
- circulates new or fresh life energy to all the organs in the body
- helps in the removal of toxic energy and waste from the body

What is physical Yoga?

Yoga means *union*, and physical Yoga is a practice of Yoga postures (*Asanas*) to build stamina, tone the body, soothe the mind, increase harmony, and step further into spirituality. A daily practice of 20–60 minutes with multiple iterations of sun salutation, or *Surya Namaskar*, is recommended to achieve the following benefits:
- improve flexibility and muscle strength
- decrease stress, increase joy and peace of mind
- help in weight loss
- improve bone health and support the spine
- increase blood flow, lower blood pressure and blood sugar
- improve sleep
- prevent digestive issues and blockages
- increase inner strength and self-esteem
- build self-awareness and encourages spirituality
- increase self-care and inculcate kindness and compassion for others

There are suggestions about the Yoga practice implemented by the three Doshas:

Vata:

- Practice at a slow and steady pace with gentle movements.
- Have a regular daily practice to prevent any stiffness in the joints.
- Do multiple repetitions and hold the poses for a shorter time to avoid exhaustion.
- Increase inhalation with each pose.
- Be focused and present during the practice.
- End the session with the relaxing corpse pose *or Savasana*.

Pitta:

- Change your focus to the body to help ease you away from your incessant thoughts.
- Immerse yourself in the present moment during the pose to self-heal.
- Make the exhalation deeper and release any negative emotions.
- Do chest and back opening postures.
- Do your practice either early in the morning or late in the evening (during the cooler parts of the day).

Kapha:

- Make your practice regular and intense.
- When you are ready to release a breath, take one more breath cycle.
- Take a pause between inhalations and exhalations.
- Challenge yourself each day as your practice progresses and keep an upward view.
- End your practice with a relaxing pose such as *Savasana*.

What is aura?

Everything in the Universe emits energy in a radiation pattern that is known as *aura*. The aura is in the form of an oval shape extending out from the body, anywhere from a few centimeters to a meter, and this energy light consists of the seven colors of the spectrum, extending above the head and below the feet. The variation in aura is based on each individual's life force, or *Prana*; strength and glow, or *Tejas*; and immunity, or *Ojas*. As one grows spiritually, the auric energy light expands farther outward.

What are Chakras?

The body has about 114 energy circles, or *Chakras*, and 72,000 energy channels, or *Nadis*, in the body. There are seven main chakras along the spinal cord, or the *Sushumna* channel (however, in *Pranic healing*, there is the idea that there are more than seven primary chakras). Each main chakra is depicted as a lotus flower with a different number of petals and a different color, and embedded within is a seed or *Beej* Mantra. We experience the rise in energy in our body from the root (lowest) to crown (highest) during the healing process.

The seven main chakras affect us on physical, emotional, and psychological levels. On a physical level, the chakras are associated with the endocrine glands in the body; namely:

- *Mooldhara* or **root chakra:** adrenal gland
- *Swadhishthana* or **sacral chakra:** reproductive glands
- *Manipura* or **solar plexus chakra:** spleen and pancreas
- *Anhata* or **heart chakra:** thymus gland
- *Vishuddha* or **throat chakra:** thyroid and parathyroid
- *Ajna* or **third-eye chakra:** pituitary
- *Sahasara* or **crown chakra:** pineal gland

As stated above, each chakra contains a *Beej* Mantra whose sound is healing to the area of the body to which it is associated. Initially, it is advised to state these mantras slowly in order to experience their vibrations:

- **Root chakra:** LAM
- **Sacral chakra:** VAM
- **Solar plexus chakra:** RAM
- **Heart chakra:** YAM
- **Throat chakra:** HAM
- **Third-eye chakra:** OM
- **Crown chakra:** OM or silence

The colors, meaning, and impact of each of the seven main chakras are illustrated below:

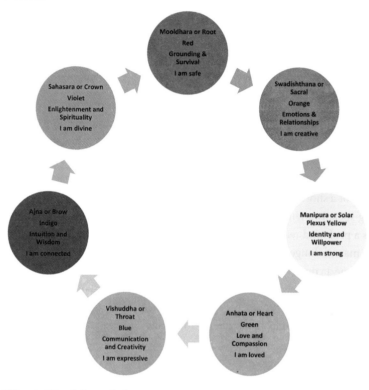

What is *Kundalini Shakti*?

Kundalini Shakti (life force power) is divine energy that is dormant at the base of the spine in the root chakra and is also known as the coiled serpent. It is the essence of life. The initiation of the awakening of Kundalini Shakti is by being aware of oneself.

During the experience of Kundalini rising or awakening, it feels like a streak of fluidlike light that flows through the *Nadis* (energy channels) and up the *Sushumna* (spinal column), passes the chakras, and cleanses blockages, as it rises to the crown chakra to merge with the *Supreme* spark. It involves a combination of various intense feelings—erotic (a sexual release), blissful, and sometimes intense anger. All current and past-life negative energies are eradicated, and the individual takes a step closer to his/her true nature.

Directly after this experience, it is possible that you could feel varying symptoms—becoming very emotional or waking up randomly at night. There is sudden realization of what does or does not work in your life, and synchronicities begin to appear in your daily life. Most importantly, there will be a heightened inner need to be of service to humanity.

It is recommended that this awakening process should be done under the benevolent grace of an enlightened guru and not by oneself, because if it is done incorrectly, it can be harmful and dangerous. This experience helps in transforming any lack of self-love or worth and forms a link with the Divine.

This purifying process brings with it a deeper comprehension of spiritual truths, which enhances your compassion to align to the energies of others. Immediately after the awakening, which helps in destroying the ego, one experiences an emotional intensity for a short period of time, as well as some discomfort, along with a feeling of being socially alienated. In due course, these emotional difficulties subside and there is a profound realization. It is possible through this transition that the experiencer may no longer be a separate individual entity (based on ego) and instead may become a conduit of the Divine.

Kundalini rising allows the experiencer to be reborn as a *goddess Shakti* who at her highest power passionately reunites with her male counterpart—Lord Shiva. It is the most life-changing experience, from which one can never go back to one's previous self.

What is Tantra?

Tantra is an ancient healing practice that allows people to meet on different consciousness planes—physical, mental, emotional, and spiritual. It is a connection between this and other levels of existence.

The word "Tantra" is known to have different meanings. It consists of two words—*Tanoti*, or to expand consciousness, and *Treyati*, or to liberate consciousness. Tantra means to weave, to expand, to spread.[7] It is when we come out of our conditioned selves that we can *reweave* into our true, original form.

Tantra aims to bring together the differing energies of *Shiva* (male) and *Shakti* (female) into oneself. It is also another way to awaken our dormant Shakti power. Tantra is both a science and a spiritual-healing journey and is often termed to be the practical aspect of Vedic tradition.

Another definition of the word "Tantra" is that it is a combination of two words—*Tattva*, or the science of cosmic principles, and mantra, or the science of the healing sound vibrations. In short, Tantra is the application of cosmic sciences with a goal for spiritual ascendancy.

A popular connotation of Tantra is that *it is a path to enlightenment*, where sexual and sensual experience is seen as a conscious meditation. It believes that sexuality is the doorway to the Divine or Higher Consciousness, and the body is the temple of God.

The experience of Tantra rejuvenates the immune system physically. In ancient times, this technique was also used for spiritual initiation—for both physiological and psychological transformation. It is a practical method for physical and spiritual healing. It has, therefore, also been known as *God's secret science* or the *secular science of ecstasy*.

In the olden days, mantras were used to focus energy, and the most popular Tantric Mantra is *Om Mani Padme Hum*, or *Hail to the Jewel in the Lotus*. It is the art of spiritualizing sexuality in order to convert negative emotions such as fear into the higher vibration of all-encompassing love, and letting go of all conditioning to allow for a complete surrender to the flow of life.

In conclusion, Tantra is a means for a union with the Divine—where you become part of the *universal cosmic energy*, thereby merging your individual energy into that of the *Supreme*.

What is *Shaktipat*?

Shaktipat is one of the highest blessings of an enlightened guru. The guru bestows his/her grace on those who are worthy of this blessing. It is the transfer of spiritual energy from the guru to the disciple through touch, the use of mantra, or transmission through the third-eye chakra by his/her benevolent gaze. This is not something that the disciple can make happen. It is imparted only after much evaluation and through grace (*Anugraha*). The guru transmits his own Higher Consciousness into the Higher Self or I AM of the disciple/recipient as an initiation process that can be done in person or from a distance.

What is *Moksha*?

Moksha in the Vedic context is what is known as *Nirvana* in Buddhism. It is reaching the highest stage in the spiritual journey—being free from the cycle of birth, or *Janam*; death, or *Mrityu*; and rebirth, or *Punarjanam*. In short, it is basically reaching the goal of *final liberation* and the path to fully return to Paramatma.

Section 9:
Understanding Your True and Unique Self

In the Vedic texts, each person has both the *Shiva* (male) and *Shakti* (female) energies. The objective is to ensure that both are balanced.

Spiritual healing refers to the path to Higher Consciousness or the I AM. In undertaking this journey, you will be able to understand your true Self and appreciate the unique qualities and skills that you have been born with. As you connect with your I AM, over time you will undergo a complete transformation and raise your energy vibration.

Why is emotional intelligence so important?

Emotional intelligence is having empathy, love, and compassion for others. Every person is primarily looking for love, respect, and connection. It also helps in raising your own self-esteem and self-worth.

In our interactions with others, when we really listen to the other, with a goal to understand rather than judge, we allow others to connect with us at a deeper level and not feel isolated. If we can be supportive to those who are going through a difficult time, we are assisting in adding hope in that person's life and improving their mental and emotional well-being.

In the absence of emotional intelligence, we will be dictated by our selfish interests and our ego, which will cause a sense of separation, conflict, and disconnection.

Why is emotional maturity so important?

Spiritual healing allows one to be in touch with one's spirit, which helps in raising emotional intelligence. In today's fast-paced world, this quality of emotional intelligence, including kindness and empathy, is essential. An added strength is having emotional maturity.

Life in general has become stressful for many due to the demands of the working world, given the economic fluctuations that have been in play in the past few years. This has resulted in mental and physical pressure for many. Each person is trying their best to cope with changing circumstances.

In such a scenario, having emotional maturity in our interactions with others makes them feel heard and acknowledged.

This is because an emotionally mature person will not spend their time and energy on blaming another but will seek to fix the issue and take full responsibility. Emotionally mature people do not lie or behave childishly during unforeseen circumstances, but they face up to reality in a calm and composed manner.

Emotional maturity is being able to manage your own emotions and use insight and understanding while interacting with others, instead of being reactive. Emotionally intelligent and mature people know how to express their own emotions without denying them or hiding them by appearing distant. This is beneficial for relationship bonding.

It is good for one to communicate how they are feeling, and they will be able to do that with ease only if the listener is supportive rather than judgmental. After all, the most crucial need for any human being is to be understood, respected, and loved for who they are.

This is especially true in schools, where a child can feel isolated or emotionally hurt by his/her classmates if they were mean through their interactions. If you find a friend feeling really upset, encourage them to speak to his/her parent, the teacher, or a counselor. This skill of emotional intelligence and understanding can be taught to a child from an early age, which in turn becomes the foundation on which he/she will build supportive personal, professional, and social relationships in his/her adult life.

How can I move toward my true authentic Self?

You are everything that is, your thoughts, your life, your dreams come true. You are everything you choose to be. You are unlimited as the endless Universe.

—*Shad Helmstetter*[1]

As we connect with our Higher Consciousness or I AM, we find ourselves to be in tune with our true, authentic Self and are able to let go of fears, anxieties, or anything that can be deemed as superficial or fake. You become intrinsically stronger, in that you do the following:

- You understand that your true Self has no anxiety, no fears, and no inhibitions.
- You take control of your life and don't hand over the rein to others. You develop your courage and take one step forward toward your dreams and goals, even if you are feeling fearful. Courage is when you are scared but you do it anyway.
- You focus on your goals and spiritual growth. You do not get distracted by what others do or say.
- You keep a distance from people who take your positive energy but cannot give you the same in return.
- You align with those who lift you up and encourage you rather than put you down or question your abilities and aspirations. There are some genuine, wonderful people in the world who know how to support and motivate others.
- You know your own needs and wants. Stay true to your dreams and work consistently toward achieving your goals.
- You don't settle in life out of fear and insecurity—know deep down that if you are doing something for the greater good, you will be supported by Paramatma.
- You let people flow into and out of your life without getting too attached or allowing it to upset you. It is said that people come into your life for a reason to teach you something, a season, or a lifetime, where they will be part of your success and failure, your ups and downs, as true friends should be.
- You understand the concept of *karma*—both good and bad—and that everything in life is a learning or karmic cycle that needs to be worked out. It is an opportunity either to change or improve ourselves or learn to let go of that which is not for our higher good. After all, we are the cocreators of our lives, and we can decide our own karma, both in the present moment and going forward.

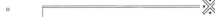

- You have complete faith and trust in Paramatma, with whom you have an intrinsic connection through your I AM. You can get downloads through a very powerful tool—your intuition.
- You are unique and valuable! Believe in yourself completely and understand your own strength. This will sustain you throughout your life.

What is the method for manifestation of our desires as a cocreator of our lives? A great many people are struggling to improve their lives—whether it is economically, personally, or both. They may perceive that they are falling short of their goals. Often, this is because they relate to their own world from a notion of lack. True manifestation can come only through the heart and soul—I AM.

The first step in changing this perspective is being thankful, which allows for the conversion of negativity into positivity. It is when we are grateful for all we have been given that we can attract more from the benevolent Universe.

In order to initiate the creative process of manifestation, send your desired request to Paramatma in solitude (to have silent communication with the Divine). It is when you are connected to your I AM that you become a cocreator in learning your lessons, understanding the bigger picture of your life, and creating plans or outcomes that bring you happiness and fulfillment based on your dharma or soul purpose. The Universe provides you with what is beneficial for your life or your spiritual ascension path, and it comes forth in divine timing.

At this stage it is best to understand a few concepts—the first is that if you do not get what you want, and it causes frustration, look within. It could be because this is what you believe about yourself—you may be holding on to a negative perception. This can be changed through a self-referral (our internal reference point is our own I AM) process.

The second concept is that often there is a delay in what we want and when it manifests. It allows us to finesse our perception—become the vision in the present—and experience it as if it has been accomplished—be completely sure that is what we really want.

The third factor is that what we wanted may have come from our ego, which may not be the best option for our life, and which is why it has not manifested as an outcome in our favor. If you do not receive an earnest wish, know that you are protected by Paramatma. If you have *Shraddha*, know that not receiving something you asked for is because it is not aligned to the bigger picture of your life or your dharma. Instead, allow yourself to be in total surrender to the flow of life with complete faith, rather than fighting it.

We then come to realize that the soul / I AM is in control, and we can see whatever comes as a blessing without any judgments—whether it is abundance or a lesson in disguise. Your internal compass / I AM is constantly guiding you, giving you insights of where you are supposed to go for your soul mission or dharma—so listen to this guidance through meditation or moments of relaxed silence.

If we take action, respond with heart-centered joy, and become fully excited to go in the direction that the soul has chartered for us, with no worry or judgment, but with complete immersion in the present moment, we will be more successful in bringing about the nonmanifested ideas, guidance, and inspiration into physical reality, as a cocreator.

In conclusion, in the words of Beverly Sills:

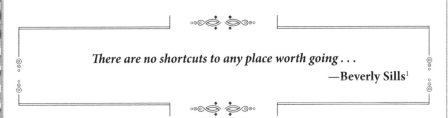

There are no shortcuts to any place worth going . . .
—**Beverly Sills**[1]

Section 10:
Maya and Enlightenment—
an Insight

What is *Maya*?

Maya means illusion/delusion or ignorance. According to the Advaita philosophy, *Maya* is a veil that hides our true nature. According to the Vedanta, the world we inhabit is constricted by time, space, and cause and effect. Our experience of it and ourselves is limited by our ego, mind, and body instead of by our divine nature—I AM.

We therefore consider this physical world as real, and by clinging to this perception, we limit ourselves—fearing the cycle of life and death along with being enmeshed in negative emotions—fear, arrogance, anger, greed, and lust.

It is only upon removing this veil of illusion *or Maya* that we can manifest our true Higher Self or true nature—that of compassion, love, service, truth, purity, and contentment. It is by surrendering to Paramatma on a regular basis through spirituality that we can have an internal awakening that moves us closer to the I AM, allowing for our true nature to emanate. It is through this self-realization process that delusion shatters and our limited perception ends, enabling us to see Paramatma in all living beings and the world at large.

The question that has often been raised is: what is the use of *Maya* in the first place?

The answer is that just as we cannot see the value of a positive scenario or outcome without having gone through a negative, stressful, and trying experience, similarly we cannot appreciate the magic of our true selves without experiencing illusion or *Maya*.

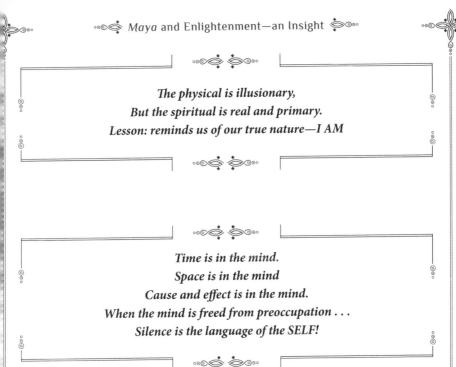

The physical is illusionary,
But the spiritual is real and primary.
Lesson: reminds us of our true nature—I AM

Time is in the mind.
Space is in the mind
Cause and effect is in the mind.
When the mind is freed from preoccupation . . .
Silence is the language of the SELF!

What is Enlightenment?

Enlightenment is the discovery of your true self—who you really are. It is only when the mind-created false self, when the ego is destroyed, that enlightenment is there. The enlightened being understands that real freedom comes from within and not through external validation.

Enlightenment is the comprehension of the truth that all negative emotions and perceptions on a day-to-day basis are transient, and once we let go of all conditioning, there is ultimate freedom—the eternal truth —*infinite consciousness* is the one sole reality. It is the formless, timeless being that is beyond time and space that is unchanging; everything else is fleeting. When we lose our false identity, we uncover that which was always there—I AM—and this is what connects us to the *Supreme* and to one another. We are all one and are from the same Source.

It is through this realization that we are able to transmute all pain and suffering into selfless love and compassion. The journey to enlightenment begins with spiritual healing as the initial step. The enlightened being gets nourishment from the *Supreme*,

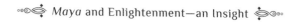

and is in complete sync with his/her inner Source. Once you see the potential value in this, you will be inspired to move toward the attainment of enlightenment and see who you really are. It is by staying in this awareness that you can live your life without anxiety and insecurity.

An enlightened being can be joyful irrespective of the circumstances or life situation and is at peace with himself/herself—allowing him/her to give compassion and love to others selflessly.

After all, an enlightened being has been awakened to pure love and connection. The true you never changes or dies but is constant—a wonderful companion, guide, and lover. In finding this pearl, you transcend all ego created emotions and trauma. You come to realize your true nature—that you are Aham Brahmasi—*I AM the Universe!*

Remember . . .
You are not your Ego . . .
You are HIGHER CONSCIOUSNESS!
I AM!
You are PURE AWARENESS!

Notes

Section 1

1. University of Minnesota's Earl E. Bakken Center for Spirituality and Healing, Regents of the University of Minnesota (2016), *Taking Charge of Your Health and Wellbeing*, https://www.takingcharge.csh.umn.edu/where-ayurveda-come-from.
2. GlobalSecurity.org (2000–2021), *Six Systems of Philosophy (Darsanas)*, https://www.globalsecurity.org/military/world/india/darsanas.htm.

Section 2

1. Gaia Herbs (2021), *Bacopa*, https://www.gaiaherbs.com/blogs/herbs/Bacopa.

Section 6

1. Helen Exley, ed., *Wisdom for the New Millennium* (Watford, UK: Exley, 1999).

Section 8

1. Vedanta Spiritual Library (2019), Celextel Enterprises, "Upanishads," https://www.celextel.org/section1/upanishads/.
2. TemplePurohit.com (2016), *Om Dyauha Shantirantariksham Shantihi*, https://www.templepurohit.com/Mantras-slokas-stotras/shanti-Mantra/om-dyauha-shantirantariksham-shantihi/.
3. Vedanta Spiritual Library (2018), Celextel Enterprises, "Tri Sloki Gita," https://www.celextel.org/other-stotras/tri-sloki-gita/.
4. Vedanta Spiritual Library (2018), Celextel Enterprises, "Vaasthu Manthras," https://www.celextel.org/other-stotras/vaasthu-manthras/.
5. Yoga Institute (2020), *Patanjali Yoga Sutra Ch 1 Sutra 20 (Parisamvad)*, https://theyogainstitute.org/patanjali-Yoga-sutra-ch1-sutra-20-parisamvad/.
6. Exley, *Wisdom for the New Millennium*.
7. LeLa Becker, "What Is Tantra Yoga?," *Seattle Yoga News*, 2016, https://seattleyoganews.com/what-is-Tantra-Yoga/.

Section 9

1. Exley, *Wisdom for the New Millennium*.

Bibliography

Becker, LeLa. "What Is Tantra Yoga?" *Seattle Yoga News*, 2016.
https://seattleyoganews.com/what-is-Tantra-Yoga/.

Exley, Helen, ed. *Wisdom for the New Millennium*. Watford, UK: Exley, 1999.

Gaia Herbs. *Bacopa*.
https://www.gaiaherbs.com/blogs/herbs/Bacopa, 2021.

GlobalSecurity.org. *Six Systems of Philosophy (Darsanas)*.
https://www.globalsecurity.org/military/world/india/darsanas.htm, 2000–2021.

TemplePurohit.com. *Om Dyauha Shantirantariksham Shantihi*,
https://www.templepurohit.com/Mantras-slokas-stotras/shanti-Mantra/om-dyauha-shantirantariksham-shantihi/, 2016.

University of Minnesota's Earl E. Bakken Center for Spirituality and Healing, Regents of the University of Minnesota. *Taking Charge of Your Health and Wellbeing*, https://www.takingcharge.csh.umn.edu/where-ayurveda-come-from, 2016.

Vedanta Spiritual Library, Celextel Enterprises. "Tri Sloki Gita."
https://www.celextel.org/other-stotras/tri-sloki-gita/, 2018.

Vedanta Spiritual Library, Celextel Enterprises. "Upanishads."
https://www.celextel.org/section1/upanishads/, 2019.

Vedanta Spiritual Library, Celextel Enterprises. "Vaasthu Manthras."
https://www.celextel.org/other-stotras/vaasthu-manthras/, 2018.

Yoga Institute. *Patanjali Yoga Sutra Ch 1 Sutra 20 (Parisamvad)*.
https://theyogainstitute.org/patanjali-Yoga-sutra-ch1-sutra-20-parisamvad/, 2020.

Glossary

Abhayanga: *Dosha*-specific herbal oil massage to loosen toxins from the tissues

Agni: Digestive fire, responsible for all digestive and metabolic processes in the body

air: One of the natural elements, and part of the *Panchamahabhutas*

Ajna: Sixth primary chakra or third-eye chakra

Ama: Buildup of toxins in the body

Amalaki: *Phyllanthus emblica*, or Indian gooseberry

Anhata: Fourth primary chakra or heart chakra

aphrodisiac: Stimulant that increases sexual desire

Artha: One of the principal aims of life, specifically wealth

asafoetida: Spice that is used to relieve stomach gas

Asana: Yoga posture

Ashwagandha: *Withania somnifera*, or Ayurvedic herb used to increase energy and reduce stress

astringent: One of the six tastes or *Rasa* in Ayurveda

Atharva Veda: The fourth Vedic text

Atma: Inner self or true self of an individual, or soul

ayu: Means life

Ayurveda: 5,000-year-old science of medicine and life from India

Ayurvedacharya: Ayurvedic doctor

Basti: Medicated enema

bitter: One of the six tastes or *Rasa* in Ayurveda

black pepper: A commonly used spice that is high in antioxidants

Brahmi: *Bacopa monnieri*, or Ayurvedic herb that sharpens the brain and improves memory

cardamom: Green cardamom (a spice used in Ayurvedic cooking), or elettaria cardamom (a digestive aid and breath freshener)

chakras: Energy vortexes in the body

Charaka: one of the principal contributors to Ayurveda and the compiler of the *Charaka Samhita*

Charaka Samhita: Sanskrit text on Ayurveda

cinnamon: *Cinnamomum*, a spice that is high in antioxidants, is anti-inflammatory, and lowers blood sugar levels

clove: Spice that is high in antioxidants and can improve liver health

consciousness: Awareness or perception or becoming awake

constitution: Qualities (physical, emotional, psychological) that are unique for each individual

coriander: Chinese parsley, a spice that has antioxidants and may promote gut health

cumin: Spice that promotes digestion and improves blood cholesterol

curry leaf: Native herb or spice of India that is high in antioxidants

dharma: One of the four principal aims of life, specifically duty

Dhatus: Tissues in the body

Dinacharya: Daily routine as described in Ayurveda

Doshas: Biological energies found in the human body and mind

earth: One of the natural elements and part of the *Panchamahabhutas*

fenugreek: Spice that is good for high cholesterol and high blood sugar

five senses: Sight, smell, sound, taste, and touch

garlic: A plant of the onion family; helps with the common cold, improves cholesterol levels, and reduces blood pressure

ghee: Clarified butter

ginger: Spice that is anti-inflammatory and has an antioxidant effect

Guggul: Ayurvedic herb that lowers cholesterol and triglycerides

Gunas: Quality or virtue

Haritaki: Ayurvedic herb that is high in vitamin C, has an antioxidant effect, and is anti-inflammatory

healing: The process of becoming healthy again

holistic: Whole, treating mind-body-spirit

I AM: Higher Consciousness God

Kama: One of the principal aims of life, specifically desire or love

Kapalbhati: "Skull-shining" breathing technique or Pranayama

Kapha: *Dosha* consisting of the elements of earth and water

Kundalini: Divine feminine energy located at the base of the spine

Kutaj: Ayurvedic herb for digestive issues and inflammation

longevity of life: Long life

Malas: Waste products in the body

Manda: Slow

Manipura: Third primary chakra or solar plexus chakra

mantra: Sacred sound or chant

meditation: Practice of awareness or mindfulness to calm the mind

mindfulness: Attention to the current or present moment, without judgment

Moksha: Salvation

Mooldhara: First primary chakra or root chakra

Mudras: Symbolic gestures

mustard seeds: Spice that contains selenium and has high anti-inflammatory effects

Mutra: Urine

Nasya: Nasal oil technique to soothe the nasal passages and reduce stress

Neem: Indian lilac and Ayurvedic herb used for stomach ulcers and skin disease, and to prevent plaque in the mouth

Ojas: Immunity

Om: Sacred sound, essence of consciousness or *Atma*

Panchakarma: Ayurvedic therapies for detoxification, cleansing, and rejuvenation

Panchamahabhutas: The five elements in nature; namely, earth, fire, air, space, and water

paramatma: Absolute *Atma*, Higher Consciousness, God

Pitta: *Dosha* consisting of the elements of fire and water

Prakruti: Unique individual constitution in Ayurveda

Prana: Life force

Pranayama: Breath control or technique

pungent: One of the six tastes or *Rasa* in Ayurveda

Rajasic: *Guna* that increases energy in the body (e.g., passion or action)

Rasa: Taste

Rasayana: Rejuvenation therapy in Ayurveda that restores the vitality of the body

red chili: A hot spice that is packed with vitamin C and antioxidants that support the immune system in the body

saffron: Expensive, fragrant spice that is a powerful antioxidant, treats depression, and is an aphrodisiac

sahasrara: Seventh primary Chakra or crown chakra

salty: One of the six tastes or *Rasa* in Ayurveda

sandalwood: Expensive spice that helps with depression and anxiety, is an aphrodisiac, and is used in religious ceremonies *saptadhatu*: Seven types of tissues in the body: *Rasa* (fluids), *Rakta* (blood), *Mamsa* (muscle), *Medha* (adipose), *Asthi* (bone), *Majja* (bone marrow), and *Shukra* (hormones)

Sattvic: *Guna* that balances energy in the body (e.g., calm)

self-realization: Understanding and fulfilling one's true potential

sexuality: One's sexual preference or orientation

Shakti: Hindu goddess, divine cosmic feminine energy

Shirodhara: Ayurvedic therapy using focused stream of herbal oils over the forehead to reduce stress and nervous tension

Shiva: Adiyogi; is nothingness and the embodiment of power

sour: One of the six tastes or *Rasa* in Ayurveda

space: One of the natural elements and part of the *Panchamahabhutas*

spice: A mix of herbs

spiritual healing: Balancing our spiritual body or soul

Surya Namaskar: Sun salutation flow in Yoga

Sushumna: Energy channel in the spinal cord

swadhisthana: Second primary chakra or sacral chakra

Swedana: Ayurvedic steam therapy

sweet: One of the six tastes or *Rasa* in Ayurveda

Tamasic: *Guna* that is negative energy in the body (e.g., lethargy, pessimism)

Tanoti: To extend, expand

Tantra: An ancient, Vedic spiritual system that enhances one's awareness to everything. It is exploring the feminine aspects of men and the masculine aspects of women (i.e., the Shiva-Shakti energies) to balance and grow spiritually. It is the weaving of energy expansion or union.

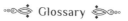

Tejas: Metabolic strength

transformation: Change or metamorphosis

Treyati: Liberation

tridoshas: Three fundamental energies that govern our physical and emotional bodies

Triphala: Ayurvedic herb that acts as a laxative and helps with weight loss

turmeric: Contains curcumin; anti-inflammatory and used for pain, depression, high cholesterol, skin problems, and liver issues

Ujjayi: Victorious breath technique or *Pranayama*

Vata: *Dosha* consisting of the elements of air and space

Vedas: Ancient Hindu script: *Rig Veda*, *Yajur Veda*, *Atharva Veda*, and *Sama Veda*

Vipaka: Postdigestion effect

Virya: Potency

Vishuddha: Fifth primary chakra or throat chakra

Yoga: means union or to yoke; to concentrate, practice to tone the physical body, calm the mind, and stay in the present moment for spiritual growth

Index

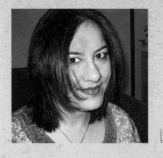

Vishnupriya Thacker is a certified holistic Ayurvedic wellness coach with a focus on mind-body-spirit well-being. She completed her training at the Institute of Integrative Nutrition with a focus on the science of Ayurveda. In addition, she gained guidance from an established Ayurvedic physician, Dr. Bapat, who in turn became the medical advisor for *A Peek into Vedic Wellness*. Her knowledge in spiritual healing was obtained through exploring various spiritual/energy healing modalities such as Vedic spiritual guidance, Reiki, chakra healing, crystal therapy, and violet flame healing. She is the founder and CEO of Vedic Synergy, an Ayurvedic wellness and spiritual-healing coaching practice in New York City. Their program offering "Rise like a Phoenix" has successfully empowered men and women to bring about a complete mind-body-soul transformation. Please visit www.vedicsynergy.com for more details. Namaste.